"The bones of the body renew themselves every seven years. With the wholesome wisdom of this book, you can help your bones provide a firm scaffold for your body."

—Mehmet C. Oz, MD, coauthor of
*YOU: The Owner's Manual* and *YOU: Staying Young*

"Annemarie Colbin is a long-time mentor of mine. *The Whole-Food Guide to Strong Bones* combines her wisdom with much common sense."

—Christiane Northrup, MD, author of *Women's Bodies, Women's Wisdom* and *The Wisdom of Menopause*

"*The Whole-Food Guide to Strong Bones* gives readers the recipe for maintaining bone health without medication. It is a must-read for anyone interested in preserving or restoring the health of their bones."

—Joel M. Evans, MD, assistant clinical professor at Albert
Einstein College of Medicine, founder and director of the
Center for Women's Health in Stamford, CT, and author of
*The Whole Pregnancy Handbook*

"*The Whole-Food Guide to Strong Bones* provides the knowledge and inspiration for maintaining a lifelong healthy skeleton. This brilliantly written book is a must-read, especially for those who may be at risk for osteoporosis."

—Carol Ellis, MD, medical director of Natural Medicine and
Rehabilitation in Branchburg, NJ

"This book by Annemarie Colbin, one of America's most respected food therapists, gives us a definitive guide to maximizing bone health as nature intended—with a balanced diet and lifestyle. Her evidence-based approach (replete with discussions of hundreds of published clinical studies) makes this book an important reference for both consumers and healthcare professionals. Plus, the recipes are fabulous."

—Woodson Merrell, MD, chairman of the Department
of Integrative Medicine at Beth Israel Medical Center in
New York City, author of *The Source*

"Annemarie Colbin is a brilliant nutritionist who has once again shown that optimal well-being can be found through living a naturally healthy lifestyle. At a time when our healthcare specialists rely too much on medications, she presents a program that relies on whole foods, exercise, and spiritual understanding. I'm happy to prescribe this book first for anyone wishing to keep their bones strong and live long."

—Stephan Rechtschaffen, MD, cofounder and chairman of the Omega Institute for Holistic Studies in Rhinebeck, NY, author of *Time Shifting*, and coauthor of *The Omega Vitality and Wellness Book*

"Movement and exercise are necessary to healthy living. But exercise is difficult if you do not have a healthy, strong bone structure to support muscle function. I look forward to giving my patients Annemarie Colbin's newest book, *The Whole-Food Guide to Strong Bones*, as it presents the most comprehensive yet understandable approach to bone health that I have encountered."

—Nancy L. Shaw, MA, MTPT, director of the Myofascial Pain Treatment Center in Washington, DC, founder of the National Association of Myofascial Trigger Point Therapists and the Shaw Myotherapy Institute

"Another classic from the mother of whole food eating, who influenced so many of us with her book *Food and Healing* over twenty years ago. Her sage advice in *The Whole-Food Guide to Strong Bones* is essential for everyone concerned about bone loss and what to do about it."

—Frank Lipman, MD, author, *Spent: End Exhaustion and Feel Great Again*

# THE
# WHOLE-FOOD GUIDE *to* STRONG BONES

## A Holistic Approach

## ANNEMARIE COLBIN, PH.D.

New Harbinger Publications, Inc.

Distributed in Canada by Raincoast Books

Copyright © 2009 by Annemarie Colbin

New Harbinger Publications, Inc.
5674 Shattuck Avenue
Oakland, CA 94609
www.newharbinger.com

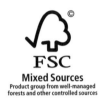

**FSC**
**Mixed Sources**
Product group from well-managed
forests and other controlled sources

Cert no. SW-COC-002283
www.fsc.org
© 1996 Forest Stewardship Council

All Rights Reserved
Printed in the United States of America

Acquired by Jess O'Brien
Cover design by Amy Shoup
Edited by Jasmine Star

Library of Congress Cataloging-in-Publication Data

Colbin, Annemarie.
  Whole foods for strong bones : a holistic approach / Annemarie Colbin ; foreword by Mark Hyman.
     p. cm.
  Includes bibliographical references.
  ISBN-13: 978-1-57224-580-8 (pbk. : alk. paper)
  ISBN-10: 1-57224-580-8 (pbk. : alk. paper) 1. Osteoporosis--Prevention--Popular works. 2. Osteoporosis--Diet therapy--Popular works. 3. Osteoporosis--Nutritional aspects--Popular works. 4. Natural foods--Popular works. I. Title.
  RC931.O73C643 2008
  616.7'160654--dc22

                        2008039812

11 10 09

10 9 8 7 6 5 4 3 2 1                                                    First printing

Part of my motivation for writing books is that I want to share useful information with my children without being always the nagging mom. I figure that if it's in a book, they can check it out when they're ready for the subject matter, and I don't have to be there. Now this motivation also applies to my grandchildren, present and future. Therefore I dedicate this book to Elijah Jaspar Dunn, Anika Luna Dunn, and Sunya Simone Lujan Gavzer, and whoever else comes along in the future, hoping they will live long, happy, healthy, and productive lives.

# Contents

## PART I
### Understanding Your Bones

CHAPTER I

CHAPTER 2

CHAPTER 3

CHAPTER 4

# Recipes

## SOUPS

## SEAWEEDS

## MINERAL-RICH GARNISHES AND CONDIMENTS

## GREEN DRINKS

## RECIPES WITH EDIBLE BONES

## DESSERT RECIPES

# Foreword

Today we are faced with unprecedented challenges for the health of our bodies and of the planet. And the most powerful tool we have at our disposal to change our health, our environment, our politics, and our economies is our fork. We have to take a hard look at our actions and our choices about food and acknowledge that the health of the human species and the health of the planet are inextricably linked. Putting six ounces of meat on our table from a commercial livestock feeding operation takes sixteen times as much petrochemical fuel and produces twenty-four times as much greenhouse emissions as growing a cup of broccoli, a cup of eggplant, a cup of cauliflower, and a cup of rice.

Industrial food production not only takes more energy but also exposes us to more harm through the processed, packaged food we are eating—through antibiotics, hormones, trans fats, high fructose corn syrup, and acidifying foods. We are consuming more animal products than our bodies need. Nutritional science teaches us that a maximum of eight ounces of animal protein a week is consistent with health, yet most people in the United States are eating eight ounces or more *a day*. It is to her credit that Annemarie Colbin has been at the forefront of the whole-foods movement for decades, and now she continues to lead the way with her groundbreaking book *The Whole-Food Guide to Strong Bones: A Holistic Approach*. In my practice as a functional medicine doctor, I see miracles daily in patients who radically improve their health by changing their diet. Applying whole foods as the primary tool of healing is the foundation of my medical practice. That is why I wholeheartedly recommend this book as a road map for mastering not only your bone health but your overall health, well-being, and aging.

Osteoporosis is a silent condition, until it isn't and you break a bone. Then it is too late. Annemarie is one of the first food writers to understand the myriad of lifestyle, dietary, and nutritional effects on our bone health and give us all the tools and wisdom to guide us through the maze of confusing nutritional advice. Among other choice bites of wisdom, we learn that vitamin D may be more important than calcium for bone health, and that we have been collectively indoctrinated that dairy is the best source of calcium and that you can't grow strong bones without it.

After twenty years of treating osteoporosis, I believe that it is a completely preventable lifestyle disease. And I believe that whole foods, exercise, and the right supplements work better than medication. Now, for the first time, we have a clear and cogent view of what makes us lose bone and what helps us keep and build bone. Optimal nutrition for bone health will completely change one of our most prevalent cultural myths: that aging equals decrepitude. Decrepitude is *abnormal* aging. You can get stronger as you get older, and *The Whole-Food Guide to Strong Bones* will help show you how.

—Mark Hyman, MD
Author of the New York Times best seller *UltraMetabolism: The Simple Plan for Automatic Weight Loss* and medical director of the UltraWellness Center in Lenox, Massachusetts

# Acknowledgments

My thanks first to Jess O'Brien, who brought me into New Harbinger and carefully shepherded this book through the process. Deep gratitude to Jess Beebe for really superb initial editing, and to Jasmine Star for her fine and precise copyediting; both helped make this book clearer and better organized. Thanks also to the sales and promotion team for their careful attention. I am happy to be part of the New Harbinger family.

I want to acknowledge a number of people for helping with a variety of aspects of the birthing of this book, including Elaine Koster, who first gave me the idea; Darwin Marcus Johnson, a graduate of the Natural Gourmet Institute, for expert help with testing a number of recipes; Mark Liponis, MD, who reviewed an earlier version of the manuscript and gave me valuable feedback on medical matters; Dr. Christiane Northrup, for her always thoughtful insights on the nature of female health; Nina Merer, for sharing her experiences in building strong bones; and Thomas Cowan, MD, and Sally Fallon, for additional information. I also want to acknowledge the many active contributors to the Botanical Medicine Listserv I subscribe to, especially Sheila Haas, Ph.D., Marie Steinmetz, MD, Katherine Falk, MD, and particularly registered dietitian and researcher Altheada L. Johnson, RD, for many contributions of research articles and commentaries on bone health, which were very helpful to me.

As always, my deep appreciation to all the students at the Natural Gourmet Institute for their interest in what I teach, and to the management and staff, who keep this institution running smoothly. It is just as amazing to see how a business born in my home kitchen in 1977 can grow into a stable and professional organization that serves its customers well as it is to see a baby grow into an independent and capable adult.

Finally, my love and thanks to my husband, Bernie Gavzer, and our children, Shana Colbin Dunn, Kaila Colbin, and Anne, Jonathan, and Adam Gavzer, as well as their respective mates, David Dunn, Michael O'Dea, Michelle Lujan, and James Campbell, for being a steady support system that keeps me feeling safe in this world.

# Introduction

*Purposeful behavior itself is often counterproductive. In seeking immediate goals (food, energy, wealth), men and women generate unending secondary effects in the natural system of which they are a part, a system which is far more complex and subtle than their information about it. "Conscious purpose, which aims toward the achievement of specific goals, does not usually take into account the circular structure of cause and effect which characterizes the universe, and this cognitive failure leads to disruption."*

—Richard Grossinger, quoting Roy Rappaport, *Planet Medicine*

Like the rest of us, I'm getting older. However, I feel very strongly that getting older is a joyful process of growing and learning; it is neither illness nor tragedy. Society, on the other hand, insists that for a woman it is both. We are bombarded with advice on how to stay young, gain eternal youth, and drop years from our appearance, often by taking various drugs and pills in an attempt to keep our bodies hormonally the same as they were during our reproductive years. We are told to shape up, lose weight, banish wrinkles, and get our faces lifted and our bodies liposucked.

I say, what for? At thirty, our sexual energy is at its peak. At sixty, our sexual energy can be at a steady and comfortable hum and, at the same time, our spiritual energy is rising. Why hold on to the past and confuse the issue? At this time in history, when we have sufficient food, shelter, and safety from predators (well, it's either the lions or the muggers, and I think city life can be as safe as life in the jungle), we can live long and productive lives and really contribute our wisdom and experience to the world. Why should we pretend to be sweet young things when we're mature men and women?

Believe it or not, this brings me to the subject at hand. Among women around the time of menopause, the subject of osteoporosis and brittle bones is a major concern. Hardly a day goes by when I don't see it mentioned somewhere or don't talk to a woman who is worried about it. More and more, osteoporosis looks like the subject of a major marketing campaign. However, it *is* true that broken hips, broken vertebrae, and broken wrists occur frequently among older people in our society, so the issue warrants attention.

When I reached menopause in the early 1990s, I refused to worry about my bones. After all, I had been paying attention to food and health for more than thirty years, and I felt that was enough. I got interested in vegetarianism in my teens and in macrobiotics in my twenties, started to teach natural foods cooking in my thirties, and then branched out into offering classes on how food affects our health and well-being in general. In the process of teaching about everything I wanted to learn, I founded a cooking school, now called the Natural Gourmet Institute for Health and Culinary Arts, and its sister institution, the Natural Gourmet Institute for Food and Health.

Because I like writing as much as teaching, I wrote two cookbooks: *The Book of Whole Meals*, published in 1979, which showed how to organize breakfasts, lunches, and dinners based on whole grains and beans, and *The Natural Gourmet*, published in 1989, with more adventuresome recipes and menus based on Chinese five element theory. In between, I wrote what I call my "think-book," *Food and Healing*, published in 1986 and reissued in 1996 in a tenth-anniversary edition. That book is my attempt to lay out a unified theory of how food affects our health, providing a basis for choosing the healthiest foods in many different circumstances and avoiding getting trapped in food ideologies that box us in too rigidly. My earlier book on the subject of bone health, *Food and Our Bones*, was published by Dutton/Plume in 1998 and went out of print in 2004. Since writing that book, I completed a doctorate in wholistic nutrition through the Union Institute and University in Cincinnati, Ohio, in 2002, which accounts for the letters beside my name.

As I paid attention to the lessons taught me by my life, my family, my children, my students, and many other people who shared and discussed their experiences with me, as well as the river of published research and information, I slowly kept changing my teaching, adding and subtracting ideas, until I came full circle and saw the benefits of many different natural foods, from both plant and animal sources. I found people who do well on vegetarian or vegan diets, and others who need not just fish but even red meat in their diets to function optimally. I found many people, including myself and my children, who do better without milk products and sugar, and others who do fine with dairy products in their diets.

What didn't vary was my view that people also need plenty of vegetables and whole grains, and that the best foods are invariably those that nature provides: whole, fresh, natural, *real* foods. I believe strongly that in a healthy diet there is no place for factory formulated, artificially colored, flavored, sweetened, or otherwise fake foods. I also found that any diet that focuses on just one of the macronutrients—protein, carbohydrates, or fats—either to emphasize or to eliminate it, sooner or later turns out to be imbalanced or insufficient. The secret, as we all know at some level, is finding the food that balances our lives.

More than anything, I believe that in order to be healthy, we need to pay attention to how we're feeling and functioning every day, not just when we get sick. Just as we keep our homes clean and our cars running with the proper amount of oil and gas, we need to keep our bodies clean inside as well as out, do mild detoxing on a regular basis, and give our bodies the proper amount of appropriate foods and fluids so we can live well and be useful and happy.

The subject of bones turns out to be immensely complex. After all, our bones are not just the hangers for our muscles and organs. They are also a repository of the many minerals that our bodies need to function properly. They are an essential part of our metabolism, keeping the pH of our blood at the right level. Indeed, they are less like stones and hard objects and more like a flowing current of nutrients and minerals. When we are in balance—a dynamic balance that involves constant movement, just like riding a bicycle—the nutrients added to and drawn out of our bones are in equilibrium and our bones remain strong. When more nutrients are extracted than are replenished, the bones become weaker.

This book looks at the entire complex system of bone health with the mission of giving you a better understanding of the topic and some practical tools for protecting your bones. Its main focus is on how food affects your skeleton, which foods weaken it, and how smart food choices can strengthen it and prevent fragility fractures. In addition, the balanced and nutritious food choices outlined in this book and featured in its recipes will help strengthen your entire body. As the song says, "The foot bone's connected to the ankle bone, the ankle bone's connected to the leg bone." Indeed, all of the bones are connected to one other and to everything else. Eating well is the best preventive medicine.

This book, then, is about keeping our bones strong with high-quality whole foods and all of their naturally occurring nutrients, along with exercise and sunlight. I hope you'll find some ideas here that apply to you, to help you remain strong for the rest of your life. Once you know the facts, your own individual course of action will become clearer. The recipes will get you started. Let's remember that, after the body dies, the bones could remain intact for millennia. If they can last that long, there is no good reason why they should weaken and break while we are alive!

# Understanding Your Bones

*One farmer says to me, "You cannot live on vegetable food solely, for it furnishes nothing to make bones with;" and so he religiously devotes a part of his day to supplying his system with the raw material of bones; walking all the while he talks behind his oxen, which, with vegetable-made bones, jerk him and his lumbering plow along in spite of every obstacle. Some things are really necessaries of life in some circles, the most helpless and diseased, which in others are luxuries merely, and in others still are entirely unknown.*

—Henry David Thoreau, *Walden*

# CHAPTER 1

# Philosophy of Nutrition: Setting Up the Point of View

*To every action there is an equal and opposite reaction.*

—Sir Isaac Newton

Before we discuss facts, we need to establish the context. I believe that having a theoretical framework, or mental model, about how things work is essential. This framework helps us understand what's going on, make predictions about what might happen next, and thereby make decisions.

We all have some sort of mental model of the world. It is cobbled together from our personal experiences, explanations offered by the social system in which we live, and additional information we gather as we grow and learn. I want to share my own viewpoint with you so that you can see where I'm coming from, and so that you can decide what mental model makes sense for you.

# MY EXPERIENCE WITH BONE HEALTH

First, let me share some of my personal observations and experiences about bone health, starting with my mother. She died in 1991, at the age of eighty-six, and was quite healthy for most of her life. Even at an advanced age, she never suffered from any illness except progressive deafness. I believe what harmed her most was a car accident she suffered at the age of eighty-one, where she was thrown from the car she was driving and given up for dead. She recuperated, but the blow to her head appeared to have started a senility process that took her downhill.

Even with the accident and several falls in the street, she never broke a single bone. She also didn't seem to shrink much as she aged, and she wasn't stooped over. Her bones may have been thin, but they didn't fracture, not even with a serious accident! Here are the aspects of her life I find meaningful in this respect:

- She had watched her diet for forty years, eating mostly whole grains and whole grain bread, vegetables, salads, and fruit, with small amounts of fish and chicken, and rarely some meat. On the whole, she avoided white flour and sugar. On birthdays and outings she would indulge in sweets, but not otherwise. Her main dietary "sin," as she called it, was coffee, which she often tried to give up but always returned to. (Not being a coffee drinker, I couldn't understand why she had so much trouble giving it up. When I asked her why she didn't drink tea instead, she dismissed the idea with a wave of her hand. "Bah," she said, "too wimpy.")

- While she did eat the occasional potato, her major sources of starch were whole grain bread and brown rice, and sometimes beans. (If this makes you think she was a woman ahead of her time, you're right. It also shows you where I came from—she was the one who taught me.)

- She never took any type of medication, either over-the-counter or prescribed. Her physician was a homeopath, whom she hardly ever visited. She felt that most of the diseases of older people are a result of the drugs and medicines they take.

- She walked a lot. Whenever she came to visit me in New York, already in her seventies, she would regularly walk forty or fifty blocks daily.

Another person who influenced my thoughts about bone health is my aunt, who was actually my mother's cousin and one year younger. She died in 1997, six months before turning ninety. She also never broke a bone as far as I know. What I saw in her was an interesting progression with weight. She was of normal weight all her life until menopause, when she put on about thirty pounds. By the time she turned eighty, she had lost that weight and more and was beginning to look really thin. Her health was quite good, and her only complaint was about her fading eyesight.

Both my mother and my aunt lived in Argentina since the late 1940s, and I returned to visit yearly from 1988. On one visit, when my aunt was about eighty-four, I noticed that she had become very thin and bowlegged, a condition she had never had before; her knees hurt on the outside, as well. She was living alone at the time and eating very little. Like my mother, she used no medications and her diet was semivegetarian, but she ate white bread and many more nightshade vegetables (potatoes, tomatoes, eggplant, and peppers—more about this later). I arranged for her to live with a caretaker, who fed her abundantly and eventually helped her put on about twenty pounds. I also instructed that her intake of potatoes and tomatoes be curtailed. Within a year, her legs had gotten stronger and the pain in her knees had disappeared.

Neither my mother nor my aunt took hormone replacements, calcium supplements or any other supplements or vitamins, or medications. They shared a disdain for pills, and I have surely inherited it. They did eat some dairy foods, both having been born in Holland, but only cheese or yogurt on occasion. They didn't drink milk regularly, or eat ice cream except as a rare treat.

More distant family members, cousins, and elderly friends did break bones on occasion. However, nobody I knew in my youth ever broke a hip. Osteoporosis wasn't a concern, and I don't recall any older women who had that thin, fragile look that is so common nowadays. However, my mother's bone strength apparently wasn't completely passed on to me, as I myself had two minor fracture episodes.

One came about when I was eleven years old and playing leapfrog with some friends at night. One of my leaps went too far, and I crashed to the ground and dislocated my right elbow. A couple of weeks later we found I had a hairline fracture and needed a cast. Fifty years later, at age sixty-one, I was marching down the street one evening in New York City, rushing toward a class I was to teach, and tripped on something in the street. Although it's usually possible recover with the other foot, in this case the other foot also tripped on the same something (I think it was a metal plate covering a hole in the street), so I went down like a tree with all my weight on my right hand. As I sat up to examine the damage, the hand looked seriously distorted. I tried to pull it straight while it was warm, but to little avail. I didn't know if the hand was sprained or broken. After some miso soup that helped me recover somewhat from the shock, I went on to teach my class—on how to keep your bones healthy, no less!—with my right hand in a sling. Then I went to the hospital.

It turned out that I had broken my wrist in what is known as a Colles' fracture, a fairly common type of break. I also had sprained many of the joints in my hand, and it took the young ER doctor about half an hour to set everything straight again. That was fairly painful and resulted in my walking around with purple fingers sticking out of my cast for a few weeks, followed by green and yellow fingers as everything healed. The fracture healed in a little over five weeks, so the cast came off quickly. The sprains took longer.

Of course I was embarrassed, as my first book on bone health had been published and I was teaching people how to keep their bones healthy. On the other hand, because it had been such a heavy and awkward fall, I felt that the fracture was perhaps inevitable and couldn't be ascribed to fragility. I suppose the entire experience fell under the category "you teach what you need to learn." Much to my chagrin, I joined the ranks of postmenopausal women who had broken a bone. Why had that happened to me? In the previous month, I think I had eaten sugar much more frequently than is my custom. But it was also the hurried way in which I walked. As Gillian Sanson says in her book *The Myth of Osteoporosis* (2003), one of the major ways to prevent fractures is to *prevent falls!* After my incident, I learned to walk slower and keep my weight more centered instead of pitching forward in a rush, which was my usual style. I did, of course, use food extensively to help me heal from this event.

There are trauma fractures, and then there are low-trauma or fragility fractures. This book addresses the latter. I am certain that what we eat can help keep us strong, prevent us from becoming weak and fragile, and thus prevent fragility fractures. But before I go into those details, I'll establish the basic theoretical framework from which I start. In order to make good decisions and choices, we need more than rules; we need a basic philosophy that directs us and is cohesive enough that our choices have the desired results. Otherwise we are at the mercy of other people telling us what to do based on *their* philosophy. Once you know where I stand, you can better make your own decisions, whether you agree or disagree with me. Follow me, then, as we take a short detour into a philosophy of life.

# THE COMPLEXITY OF LIVING SYSTEMS

Energy moves between opposite poles, and every action has its consequences. Newton integrated these concepts into the pillars of his physical laws, and many systems of thought throughout history concur. Action and reaction, up and down, night and day—these are all sets of opposites, like the two sides of a coin, and just as inseparable. You could visualize that life works like a seesaw or a pendulum. Right and wrong and yin and yang are two of the better known social constructs on this theme. For the past five thousand years, right and wrong has been the basic mode of thought in Western civilization, while yin and yang has been the foundation of Chinese thought.

The main difference between those two viewpoints has to do with judgment. Right versus wrong implies that if one part is good or right, the other automatically has to be bad or wrong, and often that is taken to mean that whatever is "opposite" must be eliminated. Yin and yang, on the other hand, are nonjudgmental descriptions. No superiority of one over the other is implied, and no destruction of one or the other is required. In fact, the two are seen as complementary and integrally interwoven. In the Chinese system, it is assumed that when one of the opposites shows up, the other isn't far behind.

When we deal with right and wrong, or good and bad, and try to eliminate whatever is considered wrong or bad, it's like cutting off your nose to spite your face. Trying to eliminate one part of the set of opposites will negatively affect the other part. This is a universal law and cannot be escaped. Here's an example: In the early 1900s, it was decided that mosquitoes were bad because they carry malaria. It was decided that mosquitoes should be eradicated, and DDT was used liberally to that end. This was action. What was the reaction? Not only did the mosquitoes die, but many birds died as well, poisoned by the pesticide. In fact, the whole earth was poisoned, and most of those toxins remain with us to this day.

Our bodies are extremely complex. John Apsley, DC, in his chapter on biogenic medicine in *The Advanced Guide to Longevity Medicine* (2001), points out that every cell in the body registers more than a million disturbances or alterations daily, all of which need to be corrected just to maintain the integrity of the system against these stresses. Multiplying that by 75 trillion (the number of cells in the body), that means that *every second of every day* the body is performing close to 870 trillion corrections! He further states that the ability to manage such a task points to a regenerative technology that can operate at near quantum speeds, that is, unlimited by time and space.

Clearly it isn't possible to manage such a complex system with linear or reductionistic thinking: one cause, one effect; or one problem, one drug. Many variables need to be addressed and accommodated. This is where a holistic approach comes in, endeavoring to look at the entire picture and attend to consequences way down the line. What does this have to do with bones? It underscores the danger inherent in going single-mindedly after a focused goal; for example, bones contain calcium, so let's take more calcium to make the bones stronger. With this approach, we may find ourselves stumbling over the law of unintended consequences because we fail to take into account the other aspects of this complex issue. We'll take a close look at this particular topic in chapter 3.

One aspect of the holistic approach is trust in the life process—trust that the body has its reasons that reason does not understand. The body's job is to stay alive day in and day out, knowing what to do with air, food, and water and how to go about repairing itself. Our bodies are born with this knowledge. It is part and parcel of each of us. When things go wrong, I believe it is important to work *with* the body's knowledge, to listen carefully to what it tells us and provide what's missing or remove what's in excess. This is what the natural healing model proposes to do: bring the body back into balance by paying attention to the law of opposites and thereby avoid triggering unexpected consequences.

Most natural healing therapies, such as acupuncture, homeopathy, naturopathy, dietary therapies, and energy medicines, look at the body as a whole system. In contrast, the conventional medical model tends to work in a simple linear fashion (if you have a headache, take a pill to eliminate the pain) rather than looking at what caused the headache to arise in the first place. That's why so many medicines actually work *against* the body, as witnessed by the list of "anti medications": antibiotics, anti-inflammatories, ant(i)acids, and the like. The all-too-common adverse effects of these drugs are often unexpected reactions of the highly complex body to the overly simplistic standard approach.

In my personal experience, the natural healing model is more accurate and has better results in dealing with disorders of function—things that the body isn't doing "right." Western medicine does a great job of dealing with structural problems and mechanical issues; in fact, nothing comes close to its ability to save lives in emergencies like car crashes, burns, gunshot wounds, and, of course, broken bones. Pharmacological drugs, on the other hand, are more problematic. *All* man-made drugs or supplements have unbalancing or adverse effects. They are a double-edged sword with both desired effects and adverse effects. Both are equal. Both count. We cannot have one without the other. When we rely on drugs for our health needs, the adverse effects must be taken into account, and expected, at all times.

No matter what your philosophy is, holistic or conventional, you'll be right in some cases and wrong in others. C. Sidney Burwell, former dean of the Harvard Medical School, has been quoted as saying, "My students are dismayed when I say to them, 'Half of what you are taught as medical students will in ten years have been shown to be wrong, and the trouble is, none of your teachers knows which half'" (Pickering 1956, 113).

For bone health in particular, numerous medications, supplements, and drugs are regularly recommended for making bones more dense, and for the fracture prevention benefits that denser bones are expected to provide. Using drugs to prevent something that may or may not happen (at least 50 or 60 percent of postmenopausal women *don't* get osteoporotic fractures) could cause adverse effects that may be worse than the problem presumably avoided. The axiom that the benefits of pharmaceutical drugs outweigh the risks mainly holds true in life-threatening situations. If the choice is between suffocating from an asthma attack and losing a little bone mass from the steroids, the choice is fairly clear. But it's an entirely different situation if the choice is between shrinking a little less and an increased risk of breast cancer associated with hormone replacement therapy. My preference is to use the natural healing model first and as much as possible, including lifestyle modifications, appropriate foods, and complementary therapies such as acupuncture, chiropractic, and massage, and only consider conventional medicine as a last resort, or in certain situations when it would be most useful.

# A PHILOSOPHY OF NUTRITION

The philosophy or theoretical framework underlying classical nutrition is based on biology and chemistry. It looks at nutrient particles and assumes a mechanistic interaction between nutrients and the body. It is reductionistic in that it reduces foods, and humans, to their constituent parts, and then studies those. In nutrition, the reductionistic model supports getting specific nutrient particles that humans are known to need. This fits in with the prevailing mechanistic model of the mainstream view of health.

Another part of the study of food is based on the discipline of thermodynamics (the study of the movement of energy and how energy instills movement). The application of the concepts of thermodynamics to digestion and absorption originated in the second half of the 1800s with the work of Justus von Liebig, a German scientist who was among those who pioneered the study of heat, oxygen, and production of carbon dioxide in humans. His work established the importance of the macronutrients—protein, carbohydrates, and fats—in energy production. After his work was widely disseminated, it became accepted dogma in Germany during the nineteenth century that these macronutrients comprised the major nutritional requirements for humans and animals. As a result, it became widely assumed that the laws of thermodynamics related to human beings and animals, and not just inert substances. This is the model that underlies the concept of calories and energy pathways. In the early 1900s, studies of human basal metabolism were conducted at the Nutrition Laboratory of the Carnegie Institution of Washington, in Boston, Massachusetts, under the direction of Frances G. Benedict. This work yielded equations that, although not error free, are still being used to calculate basal energy expenditure, or the energy required for a body at rest (Frankenfield, Muth, and Rowe 1998).

While a useful model, the reductionistic approach presents only half the picture—the trees, so to speak. It is equally as important to look at the forest, or the human being as a whole system, as well as food as a whole system. This is the holistic approach that I have used for many years. These days it is supported by complexity theory, one of the "new sciences," which states that the whole is more than the sum of its parts and that we cannot understand the behavior of the whole by studying its separate parts. Complexity science also makes it clear that the behavior of the whole cannot be approximated by adding up the behavior of the parts. For example, the qualities of water, a liquid at room temperature, cannot be inferred or approximated from the qualities of its constituents, hydrogen and oxygen, which are both gases at similar temperatures (Waldrop 1992).

Whole foods, then, contribute to the wholeness of humans because of the full complement of their nutrients, both known and unknown, and their interactions.

In making decisions about how to use foods for general health, as well as for particular conditions, I like to rely on several models. Three theoretical frameworks underlie all the work in this book. They don't always agree with one another, but I usually find that what one model doesn't cover, another one does:

1.   The standard reductionistic model of scientific nutrition: looking at individual nutrients as well as their known interactions. This gives us much good information and detail.

2.   Epidemiology and nutritional anthropology: looking at what healthy peoples around the world have been eating for generations. This gives us a broader view of the issues around bone health.

3.   The acid-alkaline model: looking at the pH balance in blood plasma. I have been using this model with great success since the early 1970s, and other authors have recently supported its validity.

Now that you have a sense of the orientation of this book and my philosophy of nutrition, let's take a look at the basic facts of how problems arise with the bones. The next chapter will take a look at what creates weak and brittle bones, the major causes of osteoporosis, and various risk factors.

# CHAPTER 2

# Osteoporosis or Fractures? Defining the Problem

*We all begin as a bundle of bones lost somewhere in a desert, a dismantled skeleton that lies under the sand. It is our work to recover the parts.*

—Clarissa Pinkola Estés, *Women Who Run with the Wolves*

Bones are built to last a long time. They decompose much later after death than the body's soft tissues, persisting for tens of thousands of years in certain conditions. Because of their durability, they have historically been used for making tools and implements. Clearly, bones are not supposed to fall apart while the body is living.

Why is it that osteoporosis has become such an issue over the past couple of decades? It apparently hasn't been a major issue before. When I checked into all the old health and nutrition books that I own, bones are hardly mentioned and osteoporosis isn't to be found in the index. But these days osteoporosis is a major public health concern. All manner of books have been written about it, and millions of women are swallowing billions of pills to keep it at bay. What has changed? What is it about our lives today that is having such a negative impact on our body's inner structure? Can this unnatural process be stopped or reversed? Will taking a few pills be enough to stop it, or do we need a whole lifestyle change? Or are we making a fuss over a natural process that needs little fussing over?

Health issues are extremely complex. They arise out of many details and variables that interact with and balance each other. If one of those variables changes, the others usually change as well. In the social communication of health concepts, however, these many variables are generally reduced to just a few sound bites, which are then presented as the only essential concepts. The others factors are overlooked and the complexity is ignored.

This has certainly happened with the issue of bone health. We face a barrage of information about the problem of osteoporosis, or the thinning of the bones—and endless marketing of so-called solutions. However, let's clarify the problem here: Osteoporosis itself is not the problem—fractures are. There are no overt symptoms of osteoporosis initially. Not only that, there are people with thin bones who don't experience fractures, and there are people with dense bones who do. We need to keep these facts in mind.

The bones that comprise the skeleton, providing structure and protecting the internal organs, are living, moving tissue. Like the shroud woven by Penelope, the wife of Odysseus, they are continuously being built up and broken down. "The bones endure nonstop makeover. The entire human skeleton is thought to be replaced every 10 years or so in adults, as twin construction crews of bone-dissolving and bone-rebuilding cells combine to remodel it," as Nicholas Wade put it in a *New York Times* article on the impermanence of the human body's cells (Wade 2005).

When the buildup of bone doesn't keep pace with the breakdown, the bone's protein structure and mineral content are diminished. If the condition continues to progress, bone mass becomes lower and lower, with increasing amounts of holes and spaces. As the bones become more porous, weaker, and lighter, the risk of fracture is thought to increase.

Historically, osteoporosis was diagnosed after a *low-impact fragility fracture*, defined as a fracture sustained after falling from standing height or less. Sometimes it was noted that the bone broke first and then the person fell down, implying that the bones had become exceedingly fragile. However, because of the new detection and measuring technology in use since the early 1990s, the definition and diagnosis of osteoporosis has changed. It is currently defined by the World Health Organization (WHO) as "a systematic skeletal disease characterized by low bone density and microarchitectural deterioration of bone tissue with a consequent increase in bone fragility and an increased susceptibility to fractures, especially of the hip, spine, and wrist" (World Health Organization 2003, xi). Note the word "disease." As bone loss occurs to everyone naturally over the years, I think the more appropriate description would be "condition." But then it wouldn't be necessary to medicate everyone just because their bones are thin, rather than because they actually break.

# WHY IS OSTEOPOROSIS A HEALTH ISSUE?

Some bone loss, between 0.5 and 1.5 percent a year, is a normal part of aging and may pose no problem. Porous bones themselves are not dangerous, nor do they cause any symptoms. The main issue is the risk of fracture, especially in the elderly. Not all fractures are caused by osteoporosis—car or ski accidents, physical assaults, and high-impact or odd-angle falls can cause fractures even in people with strong bones. Therefore, it's important to distinguish between fractures caused by high-impact trauma and those caused by fragility, either from low-impact trauma (a light fall from standing height) or simply the body's own weight (Sanson 2003). It is the latter that is a public health problem.

Osteoporosis may or may not lead to fractures; clearly it does not do so in the majority of cases. It is estimated that, in the United States, around 40 percent of white women and 13 percent of white men aged fifty years will experience at least one fracture that appears to be the result of fragility, rather than actual physical trauma at some point in their life (International Osteoporosis Foundation 2007). That means that 60 percent of white women and 83 percent of white men will not.

## Fracture Risk

According to John A. Kanis of the WHO Collaborating Centre for Metabolic Bone Diseases (2002), the following risk factors indicate osteoporotic fracture risk over and above bone mineral density measurements:

- Age

- Lack of menstruation

- Insufficient sex hormones in men

- Asian or Caucasian ethnic origin

- Previous fragility fracture

- The use of steroid drugs, which are associated with bone loss

- Family history of hip fracture

- Poor vision

- Low body weight

- Cigarette smoking

The National Osteoporosis Foundation, an advocacy organization with the mission of promoting lifelong bone health, offers the following facts and figures: In 2005, osteoporosis was responsible for more than 2 million fractures, including approximately 300,000 hip fractures, 550,000 vertebral fractures, 400,000 wrist fractures, and 800,000 fractures at other sites (2008a).

Fragility fractures in people over fifty are a public health problem because about half of those who sustain a hip fracture become temporarily or permanently disabled due to complications such as blood clots or pneumonia. Only 15 percent can walk across a room by themselves six months after their fracture, and 20 percent end up in a nursing home, a situation that participants in one study described as less desirable than death. About 25 percent may die within a year (National Osteoporosis Foundation 2008a). These fractures can dramatically alter the lives of the individuals affected. They also represent a significant health care cost. In addition, they can cause further problems for the person beyond the original fracture, such as deformities of the spine, the hunched-over condition known as a dowager's hump, and loss of height.

In both men and women, increasing age and low bone mineral density are the two most important independent risk factors for an initial fracture. Although the prevalence of osteoporosis is greater in women, mortality after fracture is higher among men. In both men and women, the incidence of vertebral fracture increases with age, although the increase is more marked in women than in men (Bonnick 2006).

The numbers are different in different countries (Colbin 1999): Reported incidences of hip fractures are highest in the United States and northern Europe, intermediate in Mediterranean and Asian countries, and lowest in South Africa, particularly in areas where people follow traditional ways of life. There are more fractures among city dwellers than among those living in the countryside, and more in current times than in the past. For example, a study published in the journal *Osteoporosis International* found that overall fracture rates were 15 percent higher among residents of downtown Rochester compared with those in the nearby rural section of Olmstead County. The same study found that the incidence of limb fractures among Rochester residents was 14 percent higher than rates documented from 1969 to 1971 (Melton, Crowson, and O'Fallon 1999; Madhok et al. 1993). Over the past forty or fifty years, the incidence of hip fractures seems to have risen significantly in a number of countries (Koval and Zuckerman 2000).

While it is believed that low bone density is a reliable indicator of higher fracture risk, the reverse is not necessarily true. In fact, one woman who came to see me for a consultation had been told she had high bone density, yet she had broken her wrist twice within a year. Dense bones may not be enough to prevent hip fractures if there are other risk factors. A study of sixty-five-year-old women by Dr. Steven R. Cummings of the University of California at San Francisco (Cumming et al. 1997) found a number of risk factors more significant than thin bones:

■ Taking sleeping pills or tranquilizers

■ Smoking

■ Having vision problems, including poor depth perception

■ Having an overactive thyroid gland

■ Being tall

■ Having a high pulse rate

■ Being unable to get out of a chair without holding onto the arms

That last risk factor is my favorite, as it allows you to test yourself easily. Simply be seated, raise your arms, and stand up. If you don't have to hold on to anything to stand up, you pass the test!

Women who had five or more of these risk factors—*regardless of bone density*—had a 10 percent chance of breaking a hip in the next five years, while those with two or less risk factors only had a 1 percent chance of doing so. In addition, it was found that smoking is a particularly noxious risk factor. Smokers were thinner, in poorer health, and less likely to walk for exercise, and had faster heart rates than nonsmokers, all factors that would increase their chances of falling and breaking a hip (Cumming et al. 1997).

---

# WHAT CAUSES OSTEOPOROSIS?

According to researchers Giorgio Cotrozzi and Patrizia Relli (1994), osteoporosis can be classified based on possible causes. There are two main categories—primary osteoporosis and secondary osteoporosis—and subcategories of each. If you've been told that you have osteoporosis or are at risk for it, consider whether any of the causes discussed below apply to you.

## Primary Osteoporosis

Primary osteoporosis occurs through natural processes of the body, including declining estrogen production and the natural loss of bone through aging. There are two main types:

1. **Postmenopausal osteoporosis (type I).** Lower estrogen levels in postmenopausal women cause a lessening of bone mass over time, starting at about 3 percent for the first year and then diminishing to 1.5 to 2 percent yearly. There are wide individual variations. Ten years after menopause some women have lost only 5 to 10 percent of their bone mass, while others have lost as much as 40 percent (Cotrozzi and Relli 1994).

2. **Senile osteoporosis (type II).** Advancing age, particularly from the seventh decade onward, brings a lower absorption of calcium from the intestine as well as decreased secretion of calcitonin, the hormone that prevents

calcium from leaving the bones. In addition, age-related osteoporosis may be exacerbated by low body mass, smoking, alcohol consumption, physical inactivity, and impaired production and metabolism of vitamin D (Tuck and Francis 2002).

## Secondary Osteoporosis

Secondary causes of osteoporosis include use of oral corticosteroids and anticonvulsants, hypogonadism or stunted sex organs, alcohol abuse, hyperthyroidism, and bone cancer. Secondary osteoporosis is responsible for vertebral crush fractures (in which the vertebrae become compressed and brittle) in as many as 55 percent of men and 30 percent of women who sustain them. Secondary osteoporosis may also be a risk factor for hip fracture (Tuck and Francis 2002). There are five main types:

1. **Endocrine osteoporosis.** This occurs as a consequence of various disorders of the endocrine glands, such as the thyroid, parathyroid, and adrenal glands, all of which are involved in bone formation. Even diabetes, a disorder of the pancreas, another endocrine gland, can cause osteoporosis because it creates problems with the metabolism of vitamin D, which helps absorb calcium from the intestines.

2. **Sedentary osteoporosis.** This arises due to bed rest or lack of physical activity, which diminishes the intestinal absorption of calcium.

3. **Malnutrition.** Bones may suffer due to a deficiency of calories or nutrients such as calcium, magnesium, various vitamins, fat, or protein.

4. **Other illnesses.** Diseases of the liver, gastrointestinal tract, or kidneys, as well as various cancers, including bone cancer, may have a secondary effect on bone formation and contribute to weakness or fractures.

5. **Iatrogenic osteoporosis.** A number of pharmacological drugs (corticosteroids, anticoagulants, antiepileptic drugs, anticonvulsants, certain diuretics, lithium, antitumor agents, and thyroid hormones) are known to cause bone loss (Cotrozzi and Relli 1994).

---

# WHO GETS OSTEOPOROSIS?

Both women and men may get osteoporosis. According to the National Osteoporosis Foundation (2008a), of the ten million Americans estimated to have osteoporosis, eight million are women and two million are men. While some risk factors are gender specific, the following apply to both sexes:

- Delayed puberty

- Excessive alcohol consumption

- Smoking

- A sedentary lifestyle or lack of exercise

- Thinness or being noticeably underweight

- Use of corticosteroids or tranquilizers

- Insufficient peak bone mass around age thirty

- Thyroid or kidney disorders

- Malignancies (multiple myeloma, bone cancer)

- Mineralization defects (osteomalacia, osteopenia)

- Gastrointestinal conditions, such as inflammatory bowel disease, cirrhosis of the liver, gastrectomy, or gastric bypass

Based on my observations and understanding of food and lifestyle, there are other significant dietary risk factors that have received insufficient attention, and which this book addresses at length:

- Eating a high amount of refined flour products and sweets

- Eating a high proportion of nightshade vegetables (potatoes, tomatoes, eggplant, peppers)

- Not eating enough vegetables, especially greens

- Not including enough good-quality fats in the diet

- Insufficient protein in the diet

You might have heard that pregnant women may lose calcium from their own bones to provide it for the developing child. Or not. Nature does not abandon mothers: According to a 2003 study, women who never had children have a 44 percent *higher* risk of hip fracture than those who did have them, *regardless of bone density*. Each additional child reduced hip fracture risk by about 9 percent. The authors conclude that the mechanism by which childbearing reduces hip fracture risk seems to be independent of the mineral density of the hip bones (Hillier et al. 2003).

Women who have borne children also appear to have a lower rate of bone loss after menopause than those who were never pregnant. This may be related to the fact that during pregnancy, women have increased levels of calcitonin, a hormone that slows down bone resorption (the release of bone minerals into the bloodstream), which protects their bones from the fetal calcium drain.

## Protein and the Bones

Both too much and too little protein can cause trouble with the bones. Some studies show that vegetarians have higher bone density than omnivores (people who eat everything, and presumably much more animal protein, but perhaps also fewer plant foods). In a 1972 study published in the *American Journal of Clinical Nutrition*, the mean bone density of seventy- to seventy-nine-year-old vegetarians was greater than that of fifty- to fifty-nine-year-old omnivores (Ellis, Holesh, and Ellis 1972). Therefore, it was generally considered that vegetarians have a lower risk of osteoporosis. Another way to interpret these studies is to note the rest of the dietary context; it could mean that the omnivores eat too many sweets and not enough greens and other plant foods. In addition, the relationship between protein and calcium may be crucial. A 1997 study found that there was an elevated risk of fracture in Norwegian women with both a high intake of protein and a low intake of calcium (Meyer et al. 1997).

However, more recent studies show a different picture. The Framingham Osteoporosis Study, which looked at people aged sixty-nine to ninety-one, found that those with the lowest protein intake had the most bone loss, and that lower intake of animal protein was also significantly related to bone loss in both the hip and the spine (Hannan et al. 2000). A study at the Bone Metabolism Laboratory at Tufts University found that a doubling of protein consumption from meat, together with a reduction of carbohydrates, not only didn't increase calcium loss through the urine, it was also associated with higher levels of bone growth factors in the blood (Roughead et al. 2003; Dawson-Hughes et al. 2004). Interestingly, soy was no better than meat in another study, where it was found that, for postmenopausal women, the substitution of soy protein for meat in a diet with average amounts of calcium didn't make any difference in the retention of calcium or in bone and cardiovascular health (Roughead et al. 2005). An earlier study showed that high-meat diets didn't create a significant change in urinary or fecal calcium or the calcium balance. There was also no significant change of the intestinal absorption of calcium during the time of high meat intake (Spencer et al. 1983).

It is time to put to rest the outdated notion that meat makes the bones weaker! (If you need additional convincing, chapter 4 includes further discussion of this topic.)

# CAUSES OF FRACTURES BEYOND LOW DENSITY

Low bone density is only one of the many risk factors for bone fracture. According to Mark Liponis, MD, a physician at Canyon Ranch in the Berkshires, "We know that many people with osteoporosis never break their hips, and some with normal bone density do. That has a lot to do with activity level, reflexes, 'padding,' sensory impairment, balance, agility, and the tendency to fall, as well as the use of sedatives or alcohol" (personal communication).

Rather than relying on bone density tests, which paint only part of the picture, perhaps the most important thing to do is to look at all of the risk factors. Test results should be considered in light of other information. When there are two or more dietary risk factors such as malnutrition, consumption of a high proportion of refined carbohydrates, and lack of vegetables or protein in the diet, as well as a sedentary life-style, these could play a role in confirming the diagnosis.

Now that you have a better understanding of osteoporosis, its causes, and the risk factors, let's take a look at how bones are formed and what they need to be healthy. This issue tends to be oversimplified with a single focus on calcium. The fact is, bone health depends on adequate supplies of many nutrients, including protein, healthy fats, certain vitamins, and a variety of minerals. Hormone levels and exercise also play a role, as does adequate hydration.

# CHAPTER 3

# More Than Calcium: What Bones Need to Be Healthy

*When illness takes the shriveling form, leafy vegetables are in order.*

—Dr. Rudolph Hauschka

To understand how to keep our bones healthy, we need to understand their structure and function. It's easy to make assumptions, especially because there has been so much marketing and propaganda about this issue. The story drummed into the public's consciousness has been that calcium is the most important element in bones and we need a lot of it, that osteoporosis happens because we can't avoid losing bone as we age, that we need drugs to keep our bones healthy, and that the only consideration in regard to food is whether it's high in calcium. In this chapter, we'll take a close look and see that while calcium is necessary, too much of it can be counterproductive, that protein plays an important role in preventing fractures, and that we can learn a lot by taking a good look at what other big-boned animals eat.

# HOW BONES DEVELOP

How bones develop from a few cells is, like life in general, quite miraculous, no matter how much we think we know about it. In the embryonic stage, bones start off as cartilage, something similar to a very firm gel, taking the same shape as the future bones. The cartilaginous skeleton is completely formed at the end of the first trimester of pregnancy. Specialized cells in the center of the long bones, in the *diaphysis*, or shaft, start actual bone formation and grow toward the ends, or the *epiphyses*, where cells also begin to *ossify*, or turn into bone. By the time a baby is born, the bones have hardened most of the way, except for a disk of cartilage between the shaft and the epiphyses. This disk, called the *epiphyseal disk*, or *growth disk*, allows the bones to keep growing until, between the ages of fourteen and twenty, the different growth disks slowly ossify and fuse the gap to halt growth.

Also during embryonic life, the center of the long bones is hollowed out to make room for the cylindrical marrow cavity. In the adult skeleton, the walls around the marrow cavity are dense, hard, and compact, and are called, appropriately, *compact bone*. The epiphyses, as well as the vertebrae, pelvis, and ribs, are less dense and contain strands of bone that crisscross haphazardly, called *trabecular bone*. Between these strands there is red bone marrow, which forms red and white blood cells. At birth the marrow in the long bones is red as well, but eventually this is replaced with yellow marrow, which consists of connective tissue, various minerals, and fat cells.

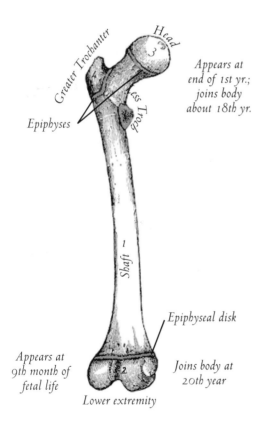

Greater Trochanter
Head
3
Appears at
end of 1st yr.;
joins body
about 18th yr.
Epiphyses
Less Troch
Shaft
1
Epiphyseal disk
Appears at
9th month of
fetal life
2
Joins body at
20th year
Lower extremity

Of course, small infant bones have to grow into child, adolescent, and eventually adult bones. In order to do that, think of this growth as a remodeling job in a house, where some parts are broken down and others rebuilt in their stead. With growing bones, this is accomplished by breaking down portions of the bone, which is done by cells called *osteoclasts*, and then rebuilding new and larger bone, which is done by cells called *osteoblasts*. It's a very complex system, and to keep it working, the osteoclasts have sacs of enzymes that, with the help of vitamin A, remove the unwanted sections. For this reason, vitamin A deficiency stunts the growth of children; as soon as it is replenished through food or supplements, growth proceeds once again.

# WHAT BONES ARE MADE OF, AND HOW THEY WORK

Bones are composed of a *collagen matrix*, a latticed protein structure that comprises about 35 percent of the bone and gives it its flexibility. This matrix is laid down first and then traps the mineral salt calcium phosphate, also known as hydroxyapatite, which makes up most of the remaining 65 percent of the bone mass and gives the bone its hardness. The bones are also the depositories of other minerals needed by the body, including magnesium, sodium, and potassium. The ability of the bone to absorb and hold on to calcium salts and other minerals is called *mineralization*.

Even though they're strong and hard, bones are not the equivalent of stones or rocks. Instead, like the rest of the tissues in the body, they are constantly moving and changing. They are continuously being built up in a process called *deposition*, or *formation*, and just as continuously being broken down, a process called *resorption*. During childhood and adolescence, this process is called *modeling* and involves removal of old bone and formation of the same bone at another site, sometimes simultaneously, to allow the bones to grow and shift in space. In adulthood, once the skeleton is set at its adult size, the same process is called *remodeling* and is more sequential, in that osteo-clasts break down old bone, and osteoblasts build new bone in that same site.

In adults, about 5 to 10 percent of bone is replaced yearly in this fashion, so that most of our adult skeleton is replaced about every ten years. From birth until sometime in our twenties, bone is built up faster than it is broken down. In young adults, this process is normally in balance; that is, deposition and resorption are equal. By about age thirty, we've generally reached peak bone mass, and from then on bone resorption is slightly higher than deposition.

Decreasing bone mass eventually creates a condition called *osteopenia*, meaning just that: a general loss of bone mass. When remodeling is abnormal and bone mass decreases but the remaining bone has normal mineralization, the condition is called *osteoporosis*. When bone mass decreases and mineralization is abnormal, the condition is called *osteomalacia*. If mineralization is defective in growing bones, causing softness and bending, the condition is called *rickets*.

# CAUSES OF FRAGILITY FRACTURES

Fragility fractures occur when there is a low-impact trauma, such as a fall from stand-ing height, when a person normally wouldn't break any bones. When a person sustains a fracture after such a minor fall, the bones are considered fragile. This happens most commonly in elderly or malnourished people with thin bones.

However, being hard and rich in calcium isn't enough to make bones resistant to fracture. Bones can be dense yet brittle and lacking in flexibility, which will cause them to break easily. The collagen matrix is crucial for maintaining flexibility and may be more essential to preventing fractures than calcium content. Consider this: If a bone is put in an acid solution and all the calcium is removed, it can be bent and twisted like a tendon. In other words, a bone with zero calcium doesn't break, *it bends* (Buckwalter et al. 1996). It's worthwhile to remember this when faced with the relentless marketing of calcium for bone health.

On the other hand, a dense, high-calcium bone with a diminished collagen matrix can break with slight pressure or shatter under a sharp blow. Think chalk. For this reason, tests that measure bone density often don't accurately predict the risk of fracture. Some people with demonstrated low bone mineralization never break a bone, in spite of repeated falls; that's because their bones are *flexible*. On the other hand, sometimes people with high bone density break their bones anyway. Unfortunately there is no simple test to determine the strength or flexibility of the collagen matrix (Snyder et al. 2006).

Of course, the simplest test to check your risk of fracture can be performed by anyone and often is: If you fall and don't break a bone, your bones are good and your risk of fracture is low. Have you tried it yet?

Obviously anyone can break a bone due to falling from a height or sustaining a high-impact trauma, such as being in a car crash or getting trampled by football players. That kind of fracture has nothing to do with osteoporosis.

# BONES AS NUTRIENT BANKS

Bones contain about 99 percent of all the calcium in the body (bound with phosphorus, remember); the remaining 1 percent is mostly in the blood and the cells. About 85 percent of the body's phosphorus is also stored in the bones. In addition, our bones store between 40 and 60 percent of our body's total sodium and magnesium.

Because our bones are a reservoir of numerous minerals that our bodies need for day-to-day functioning, the remodeling process is essential to our general health, as it liberates these minerals to be used as needed and allows them to be replaced again. Our bones, in fact, act a little like a bank. Nutrients come and go as a continuous flow of "income" and "expenses." Calcium is the major element in this flow and deserves a good look.

# THE ROLE OF CALCIUM

Calcium is the most abundant mineral in the body and is absolutely essential for many physiological functions, as it is one of the major electrolytes. As such, it is used throughout the body in electrical communications and functions such as nerve transmission, muscle contraction and growth, general metabolism, heart function, blood clotting, and various enzyme and hormone functions. The correct amount of calcium in the blood is vital for survival, much more so than levels in the bones. That's because insufficient calcium and magnesium in the blood increases its acidity (lowers its pH), which affects electrical signaling, and may, among other things, then affect the beating of the heart (Rylander et al. 2006).

## How Calcium Travels

The major sources of calcium are the foods we eat. Food is broken down in the stomach and duodenum, the upper part of the small intestine, and becomes a partially digested mass called chyme. Then, as the chyme travels through the remaining twenty or so feet of the small intestine, minerals are absorbed through its walls straight into the bloodstream with the help of vitamin D. Interestingly, absorption of calcium from the intestine is on average only about 150 milligrams (mg) per day, since some calcium is secreted back into the intestine as part of its digestive juices. The extracellular fluid (the fluid that bathes the body's cells) must maintain a constant level of calcium for normal cell function, and there also must be sufficient calcium inside the cells for their metabolic activities. Some calcium also remains unabsorbed in undigested parts of the food and is excreted through the bowels.

Once in the blood, calcium is one of the electrolytes that help keep the blood pH stable. Whatever calcium isn't needed in the blood can go straight to the bones and be deposited there for storage. When the blood pH becomes low, parathyroid hormone activates bone resorption, liberating calcium for maintaining the functions of the muscles, nerves, heart muscle, and blood. So as you can see, the ability of the body to manage calcium flow in and out of the bones is indeed crucial to our survival.

Excess calcium that doesn't go back into the bones is sometimes excreted by the kidneys. Many years ago, I had a student who regularly developed calcium deposits in her ureter (the tube that brings urine from the kidneys to the bladder), which meant she had to go to the hospital regularly to have it reamed out. Once they put a tube from her kidneys to her bladder to allow the urine to flow while her ureter healed; within a day or two there were calcium deposits in the tube. Her doctors were stumped. I asked her, "How much milk do you drink?" "Oh," she replied, "about a quart a day." "Even in the hospital?" "Yes." "Did anyone inquire about this?" "No." I suggested that she totally stop drinking milk. When I saw her a few years later, she'd had no recurrences of the problem, had a new baby, and was in fine health. Granted this is an unusual case, but it illustrates what can happen with too much of a "good thing."

## How Calcium Travels

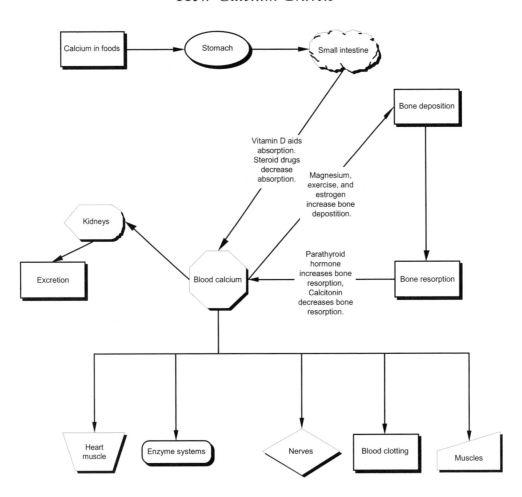

Continuing with our analogy between the bones and a bank, we need all kinds of helpers (tellers, accountants) to get the money (calcium) from here to there, and we may encounter all manner of systems that check excessive growth. Also, it's important to realize that interfering with this process with pharmacological drugs that prevent resorption means that the bank account becomes frozen, so we won't be able to pay the rent; in other words, the body won't have access to the calcium and other minerals in the bones to keep the blood pH at the right level.

What is the main helper element that keeps this input and output system moving? It's activity. Movement, walking, and the influence of gravity all help the deposition of calcium in the bones. It's well-known that sedentary living, being bedridden, and weightlessness (as experienced by astronauts in space) all contribute to the loss of bone mass. Immobility prevents the deposition of calcium salts, so the process of mineral resorption slowly depletes the available bone mass. In other words, "Use it or lose it!"

## Sources of Calcium

Thanks to skillful marketing, everyone knows that milk products are a major source of calcium. If you're allergic to dairy or just feel better without it, you may worry about getting enough calcium. Don't worry; there are plenty of other sources of calcium that may actually be easier for your body to absorb. You can get your calcium from the same source as big-boned animals like horses and the elephants get theirs: leafy greens. I know most people think that won't provide enough calcium, but the amount they do provide is sufficient for bone health and therefore is enough.

The following plant foods contain plenty of calcium that is highly bioavailable, almost twice as much ounce for ounce as in milk products and even calcium-fortified foods and beverages: cauliflower, watercress, parsley, Brussels sprouts, rutabaga, kale, mustard greens, bok choy, broccoli, and turnip greens. (Spinach and chard also contain calcium, but due to the presence of oxalates, or oxalic acid, which bind the calcium, it is generally less available.) Although slightly less bioavailable, calcium is also abundant in almonds, sesame seeds, pinto beans, and sweet potatoes. Other good sources include seaweeds, often used in Japanese dishes such as sushi rolls (nori) and miso soup (wakame). Mineral waters are also often a good natural source of calcium.

Among the animal foods rich in calcium are oysters, soft-shell crabs, and especially food preparations including edible bones, such as small fish with bones (sardines and anchovies), and mineral-rich stocks made with bones (Whitney and Rolfes 2005; Fallon 1995).

In a meal that has many different sources of calcium, such as beans, greens, and seafood, for example, you will end up getting enough even if each separate foodstuff is not a major source of the mineral.

---

# BEYOND CALCIUM

The human body is a very complex system. It is a whole much larger than the sum of its parts. And most importantly, all of the parts work together in synergy, and all depend on one another for proper function. Being but one element in this complex system, calcium needs many other nutrients to balance it in order to be useful to the bones.

As we know, a common misconception is that a high intake of calcium is by itself the main element required for bone health and the prevention of fractures. D. Mark Hegsted, Ph.D., formerly of the Nutrition Department of the Harvard School of Public Health, clearly disputes this myth:

> Worldwide data raise serious questions about the relation between calcium intake and fractures. A large proportion of the world's population consumes low-calcium diets and, although quantitative data on the fracture rate in such populations are limited, it is obvious that these populations do not have excessive rates of fractures as would be expected if calcium requirements

were far above their usual intake. Good data on the association of fracture rates with calcium intakes are available from Japan and clearly show that Japanese women have both less bone mineral and far fewer fractures than do American women. It seems obvious that whatever the importance of calcium intake and bone mineral content may be, other important factors must be involved in determining the susceptibility to fractures. (2001, 572)

And then he asks a very good question: Why do populations who consume low-calcium diets have fewer fractures than do people in Western societies, who consume high-calcium diets?

Balance is the key, which means that focusing on a single element is counterproductive and causes imbalance. All of the elements have to work together harmoniously, without any of them in either deficiency or excess. This relates to what I like to call the "three bears rule": Too much is no good and too little is no good; we need to get it *just right*. Too much supplemental calcium can actually cause problems. For example, one study found that it increased the risk of stroke and cardiovascular disease (Bolland et al. 2008).

Beyond calcium there are many other nutrients and factors that have a crucial influence on how bone is formed and resorbed. Here are some of the major ones:

- Vitamin D helps absorb calcium from the intestines.

- Phosphorus is essential for proper mineralization of bones and teeth.

- Vitamin A helps in the bone growth of infants and children.

- Protein and vitamin C stimulate collagen matrix formation.

- Magnesium increases calcium absorption from the blood into the bones.

- Vitamin K is necessary for blood clotting and maintaining good bone density.

- Healthy fats are required to absorb fat-soluble vitamins, such as D and K.

- Strain, stress, exercise, and movement increase bone deposition.

Let's take a closer look at each of these factors, as well as the role of hormonal influences, water intake and hydration, and sodium.

# VITAMIN D

One of the main elements for bone health is vitamin D, which is actually a hormone. Vitamin D is made by the body when sunlight hits the cholesterol in the skin. It helps absorb calcium from the small intestine, so it's essential for bone formation. It also aids in the assimilation of phosphorus. Interestingly, the production of this vitamin/hormone ceases when the body's calcium needs are satisfied, so the rest of the calcium in the intestines is simply excreted (Seely 2002).

There are two forms of the vitamin: $D_2$ (also known as ergocalciferol) and $D_3$ (also known as cholecalciferol). The former is found more in plants, the latter in the tissues of animals (including humans). Throughout this book, mention of vitamin D usually refers to vitamin $D_3$. Be aware that supplemental vitamin $D_2$ is considered one of the more toxic vitamins, so it should only be taken with great caution.

Because vitamin D is fat soluble, there must be a sufficient amount of good-quality fats in the body to store this "sunshine vitamin." Mainly for this reason, low-fat diets don't support healthy bones. In Ayurvedic dietary philosophy, there is a saying that "good fat makes good bones." More on fats later.

Awareness of vitamin D's important and multifaceted role in health is growing. This important nutrient is now known to protect against many health problems, including the following (Masterjohn 2006):

- Rickets and osteomalacia

- Hypocalcemia (deficiency of calcium in the blood)

- Convulsions, tetany, and heart failure in newborns

- Osteoporosis

- Cancer

- Heart disease

- High blood pressure

- Obesity

- Arthritis

- Mental illness

- Chronic pain

- Muscular weakness

- Radiation poisoning

- Diabetes

- Multiple sclerosis and other autoimmune diseases

# Sunlight and Vitamin D

Through its action on the cholesterol in our skin, sunlight is our main source of vitamin D. This is how it works: The action of sunlight on a form of cholesterol in skin oils prompts the formation of a precursor, previtamin D, which then is absorbed through the skin back into the body. It goes to the liver for initial processing, and then to the kidneys, which finally produce the active form, vitamin $D_3$. The entire process takes about thirty-six hours.

Given enough sunshine, people need no vitamin D from foods. In the absence of enough sun, foods need to make up the lack, or one can resort to supplementation. The body's production of vitamin D can be as high as 20,000 international units (IU) with full-body sun exposure in areas around the equator; this amount is received in the time required to develop a very slight redness. The physiological reason why people are so avid about getting a tan in the summer may be because they feel a deficiency of vitamin D, and tanning, or exposure to ultraviolet light, is a way to replenish body stores of this important substance. The body can accumulate vitamin D and store significant reserves in the liver, spleen, bones, and brain, which can then be used up slowly during the darker months. This is helpful in geographical areas where there is little sun in the fall and winter. It's unfortunate that sunlight on the skin is now considered a health hazard; if that were a correct assessment, our species wouldn't have survived on the earth as long as we have without sunscreen.

Getting vitamin D naturally, from exposure to sunlight whenever possible, *while avoiding sunburn*, is most preferable. This allows the body to make what it needs and no more, thereby avoiding toxicity. Remember, vitamin D is fat-soluble, so you must have sufficient good-quality fats in your diet to be able to store it for the winter months.

According to Michael F. Holick, director of the Vitamin D, Skin, and Bone Research Laboratory at Boston University Medical Center, about 30 to 40 percent of the people who get hip fractures are deficient in vitamin D. In an interview published in *Nutrition Action Healthletter*, published by the Center for Science in the Public Interest, he points out that regardless of the amount of calcium consumed, vitamin D deficiency accelerates bone loss and increases the risk of fractures (Liebman 1997). In a paper published in the *American Journal of Clinical Nutrition*, Dr. Holick points out that a deficiency in vitamin D, known to cause rickets among children, also worsens osteoporosis among adults and can cause osteomalacia, a bone disease accompanied by considerable pain (Holick 2004).

To prevent vitamin D deficiency, he recommends walking with your face, hands, and arms exposed to the sun two or three times a week, for about half the time it would take to get sunburned—between ten and twenty minutes depending on your skin tone, the season, and the distance from the equator. Most importantly, Dr. Holick recommends this exposure to the sun be *without sunscreen*, as sunscreen interferes with the production of vitamin D. Sunscreen with an SPF (sun protection factor) of 8 allows only 5 percent of normal production of the vitamin, while with an SFP of 30 virtually none is produced.

This is important to note because as many as 75 percent of the people who seek osteoporosis advice are considered deficient in vitamin D, meaning they have less than 30 ng/ml (nanograms per ml) in the blood (Guardia et al. 2008). There is growing suspicion among some health professionals that this is due to the liberal use of sunblock, along with our indoor lifestyles, focused on work, computers, video games, or TV. Going outside may not help us much if we go from the house to the car to the office to the mall to a restaurant. Even children are deficient, as they so seldom play outdoors anymore—and if they do, their parents carefully slather them with sunscreen before they leave the house.

Katherine Falk, MD, a psychiatrist in New York City who regularly checks her patients' vitamin D levels, found that everyone she tested had a very low level, except for a young woman who regularly went to a tanning salon, who tested normal to high (personal communication). Maybe we should all go back to getting nice tans! Authors of a study in the Netherlands believe that while public information should warn against too much sunbathing, it also should encourage regular, if limited exposure to the sun's healthful, warming rays (van der Rhee, de Vries, and Coebergh 2007). Another study, this one from Germany, makes the same point: There should be enough sun exposure for health, but not so much as to burn the skin, which could provoke skin cancer, and dermatologists should be aware of this (Reichrath 2006).

## What It Does and How Much We Need

According to Walter Willett, professor of epidemiology and nutrition at the Harvard School of Public Health and one of the principal investigators of the Nurses' Health Study II, which has followed more than 100,000 registered nurses since 1989, high vitamin D intake reduces the risk of hip fractures and is associated with higher bone density (Feskanich, Willett, and Colditz 2003). Sufficient vitamin D is also thought to prevent falls, which are a major risk for fractures (Jackson et al. 2007). Along these same lines, a review paper in the *Journal of the American Medical Association* determined that a daily intake of 400 IU or more resulted in a 20 percent reduction in the likelihood of being injured in a fall. This may be because vitamin D appears to strengthen the thigh muscles, which are crucial for gait and balance (Bischoff-Ferrari et al. 2004).

Optimum levels of vitamin D in the body are clearly associated with protection against a number of common diseases, including diabetes, osteoporosis, osteoarthritis, hypertension, cardiovascular disease, metabolic syndrome, depression, multiple sclerosis, and cancers of the breast, prostate, pancreas, and colon (Vasquez, Manso, and Cannell 2004). A study at the Meir Medical Center at Tel-Aviv University in Israel found that vitamin D is a biological inhibitor of inflammation and can be very useful in treating and even preventing autoimmune disorders such as multiple sclerosis and type 1 diabetes (Arnson, Amital, and Shoenfeld 2007).

Sun exposure has been found to have an inverse relationship with numerous other cancers (more sun, less cancer), including cancer of the colon, prostate, uterus, stomach, esophagus, thyroid, and bladder. Results of one population study suggest that maintaining adequate vitamin D levels is more critical for limiting the progression of tumors than for preventing their onset (Boscoe and Schymura 2006). Interestingly, it is thought that vitamin D may also protect against cutaneous melanoma of the head and neck, which tends to develop later in life (Vollmer 2007). You'd think that those cancers would develop *earlier*, because of sun exposure, wouldn't you? But it seems they don't.

Thomas Perez, a health science researcher and administrator with the U.S. Food and Drug administration, offers a contrary point of view: that the causal relationship may work the other way around. Rather than vitamin D deficiency causing some diseases, these diseases may cause the deficiency (personal communication).

How much vitamin D do we need? The 1997 recommendation from the Institute of Medicine (within the National Academy of Sciences) is about 400 IU daily, or 10 micrograms (mcg). According to a 2004 review study in the journal *Alternative Therapies in Health and Medicine*, the original upper limit for safe intake of vitamin D was set too low, at 2,000 IU per day, or 50 mcg. It is now believed that the physiological requirement may be as high as 2,400 IU, or 60 mcg, daily (Vasquez, Manso, and Cannell 2004).

As with practically all other nutrients, vitamin D does not act alone; it has interactions with vitamins A and K. In fact, some researchers postulate that vitamin D toxicity may result from a relative deficiency of vitamins A and K. The former is needed for the hormonal activity of vitamin D, and the latter is needed to help activate the proteins resulting from the physiological response to them. Also, it is thought that vitamin A toxicity may relate to a deficiency in vitamin K. In other words, those three are closely intertwined and must be considered together (Masterjohn 2006). In the Nurses' Health Study, it was found that women with high levels of vitamin D but low levels of vitamin K had a greater risk of hip fracture than those with low levels of both (Feskanich et al. 1999).

Be aware that mineral oil can destroy vitamin D in the intestines. Therefore, when used as a laxative, this substance can interfere seriously with calcium metabolism.


## Food Sources

Vitamin D from food sources is absorbed through the intestines in the company of essential fatty acids. Good dietary sources of vitamin $D_3$ are wild ocean fatty fish such as mackerel and wild ocean salmon (make sure to eat the skin!), as well as caviar or fish eggs. Try salmon caviar or the Greek *taramasalata*; two or three servings per week are quite sufficient. Cod liver oil, of course, is the classic source of vitamin D that has been used for generations in northern Europe, where there is little sun, especially in the winter months, and therefore much less opportunity to obtain this nutrient from sunlight. In addition, vitamin D precursors, known as ergosterols, are present in plant foods and leafy greens; parsley is a particularly rich source. Ergosterols are also abundant in shiitake mushrooms; 1 ounce (after soaking and cooking) of dry shiitake mushrooms contains about 46 percent of the recommended daily amount of vitamin D for a fifty-five-year-old woman. There may also be significant amounts in other wild mushrooms (Outila et al. 1999). A study of the Japanese diet found that about 90 percent of its vitamin D content comes from wild ocean fish, and some 4 percent from mushrooms (Nakamura et al. 2002).

## Supplemental Sources

Vitamin $D_3$ can be made synthetically by ultraviolet light irradiation of a derivative of cholesterol. Vitamin $D_2$, or ergocalciferol, has a different synthetic form. The vitamin D added to milk, a practice begun in the 1930s to prevent rickets, can be either of those two synthetic forms. Consumers may feel they're getting enough vitamin D if they drink fortified milk. However, according to studies published in the *New England Journal of Medicine* in 1992 and 1993, out of ten samples of milk, seven had less than 80 percent of the amount listed on the label, five didn't even have 50 percent, and 14 percent of samples of skim milk had no vitamin D at all (Holick et al. 1992; Chen et al. 1993).

An excess of supplemental vitamin D—now considered to be serum blood levels in excess of about 80 mcg per milliliter of blood—can be seriously toxic, causing calcification of soft tissues and of the walls of the blood vessels, heart tissues, lungs, and kidney tubules, a condition known as hypercalcemia. In one unusual case in New England in the early 1990s reported in the *New England Journal of Medicine*, some infants developed this condition from excess vitamin D fortification of milk through a measuring error at the dairy. Instead of the standard 400 IU per quart, the concentration in some samples went from undetectable to as high as 232,565 IU per quart. Hypercalcemia is a serious condition, as it can result in calcium deposits in the soft tissues and organs, and arteriosclerosis, sometimes within a day or two of exposure. Tragically, in the case of these infants it caused hardening of the cranial bones and premature closing of the fontanel, which led to irreversible brain damage (Jacobus et al. 1992).

However, according to Mariana Markell, MD, associate professor of medicine at SUNY Downstate Medical Center, hypercalcemia from vitamin D ingestion is rare in the absence of other conditions, and given that many of us are deficient in vitamin D, it's even rarer than one might predict (personal communication).

Here's the bottom line: If you can, get your vitamin D from sunshine, *without burning*. Consider a tanning salon if it isn't possible for you to spend time out in the sunshine. Depending on your skin, the amount of exposure needed may be anywhere from ten to thirty minutes. Some very fair people will react to the sun quickly, whereas darker-skinned people may take longer. This approach allows your body to make what it needs, and no more, thereby avoiding any risk of toxicity. Food sources such as fatty fish, mushrooms, and parsley can be consumed liberally. And finally, in the case of demonstrated vitamin D deficiency together with other medical conditions, careful supplementation, such as with cod liver oil, under the care of an enlightened medical practitioner is a viable option.

# PHOSPHORUS

Phosphorus is the second most abundant mineral in the body. As mentioned, it is a major component of bones, together with calcium, in the form of calcium-phosphate salts. In addition, it plays an important role in every cell in the body, where it helps maintain the acid-alkaline balance (discussed in chapter 4). It also supports the function of the B vitamins as well as some enzymes. Importantly, it is a component of the phospholipids, which carry the fats needed for energy metabolism through the blood, and help maintain the integrity of all cell membranes.

Insufficient phosphorus prevents the body from creating the necessary calcium salts and weakens the bones. Excess phosphorus in the form of phosphoric acid (found mainly in soft drinks, preservatives, and meat) can stimulate the release of calcium from the bones and thereby weakens them as well (Whitney and Rolfes 2005).

Phosphorus is abundant in the food supply, particularly in animal protein, especially liver, but also in sunflower seeds, almonds, and beans. While soft drinks are a common source of phosphorus in the form of phosphoric acid, this substance blocks the absorption of both calcium and magnesium in the intestines, so it can directly contribute to the formation of brittle bones (Fallon 1995). In addition, I would consider them a very poor source of phosphorus because of the other ingredients they contain. Deficiencies of phosphorus are unknown. Excessive amounts have been associated with calcium deposits in soft tissues and kidneys.

# VITAMIN A

Vitamin A, which is fat-soluble, is required for bone remodeling. It can be found abundantly in animal foods and certain plant foods. The best sources of preformed vitamin A, or retinoids, are the fats and organs of healthy animals, including liver, fish liver oils, wild ocean fatty fish, and butter from cows that have been grazing on green grass. (Cows that are fed grain don't have much vitamin A in their milk, hence the custom of fortifying milk with that vitamin.)

Numerous plant foods carry the precursors for vitamin A, known as the carotenoids. The carotenoid with the most vitamin A activity is beta-carotene, an antioxidant and the phytochemical that gives fruits and vegetables their yellow, red, and orange colors. It is also found in leafy green vegetables. Beta-carotene is converted to vitamin A in the body.

As vitamin A is fat soluble, it can be stored in the body. Therefore, it's possible to accumulate so much that it becomes toxic, either by supplementation or by eating a lot of the foods containing it, such as daily use of chicken liver spreads or, should you have the opportunity, elk or polar bear liver. Toxicity may include bone problems such as higher fracture risk, birth defects, and cell damage. Toxicity from plant-derived beta-carotene is more rare, and much less dangerous. It may manifest simply as an orange hue in areas of the body with lighter skin, such as the palms of the hands; lowering or ceasing consumption will reverse the condition. Excess vitamin A from supplementation, on the other hand, may cause more problems, including a higher rate of hip fractures (Lim et al. 2004) and also of spine and wrist fractures (White et al. 2006).

# PROTEIN AND VITAMIN C

Either too much or too little protein can cause trouble with the bones. For quite some time, it was thought that protein weakened bone. However, the formation of collagen is dependent on sufficient protein in the diet, as well as vitamin C, which stimulates the enzymes that form collagen and connective tissue. A deficiency of either one could weaken the bone matrix, interfering with its ability to hold on to calcium salts.

Sufficient protein from animal sources is now considered essential for a reduced risk of fracture (Wengreen et al. 2004). Protein is found most abundantly in meat, poultry, fish, eggs, beans, nuts, and seeds, and in lesser amounts in whole grains. Vegetarians need to consume enough protein from beans and nuts *in each meal* to protect their bones (and also make sure to get enough calcium from plant sources, such as greens). Interestingly, while a study of people on a raw food vegetarian diet found it to be associated with low bone mass at clinically important skeletal regions, it didn't reveal any evidence of other risk factors (Fontana et al. 2005).

Vitamin C, required for collagen synthesis, is found in all fruits and vegetables. However, it does break down quickly in the presence of heat or oxygen, so the fresher the food the better. People who eat carelessly, focusing on packaged and processed foods and refined carbohydrates and ignoring vegetables and protein, may be risking weak bones from collagen matrix insufficiency. In these cases, calcium supplements may be counterproductive; an excess of calcium combined with a lack of collagen matrix could make the bones hard and dense, but brittle, and therefore more easily breakable.

# MAGNESIUM

Magnesium is needed to stimulate the absorption of calcium into the bones (Nieves 2005). If there is a lack of magnesium, supplemental calcium may not go into strengthening the bones but instead remain in the bloodstream, perhaps contributing to various calcium deposits, kidney stones, or gallstones. Nan Kathryn Fuchs, Ph.D., a nutritionist at the Health Center in Santa Monica, California, and editor of the *Women's Health Letter*, points out that while magnesium helps the body absorb and make use of calcium, excessive calcium prevents the absorption of magnesium, and that supplementing calcium but not magnesium may cause difficulties with calcium absorption or lead to magnesium deficiency. Symptoms of magnesium deficiency include hair loss, muscle contractions or cramps, nervous irritability, tremors, disorientation, and confusion (Fuchs 2003).

You may be surprised to learn that increasing magnesium intake while *lowering calcium intake* to 500 mg per day has been shown to increase bone density (Nieves 2005). Magnesium is found in whole grains, beans, fruits, and fresh vegetables. It is refined out of sugar, white flour, and white rice, so here is another reason why these foods are counterproductive for bone health. Both sugar and alcohol cause magnesium to be excreted in the urine.

Perhaps you'll be pleased to know that one of the foods highest in magnesium is chocolate, or cocoa powder. Is this an invitation to eat more chocolate? Not really. Unfortunately, the stimulants in chocolate—caffeine and theobromine—should give us pause, as it is well established that caffeine consumption contributes to low bone density (Hallström et al. 2006). A paper in the *Journal of the American Dietetic Association* found that some people may use chocolate as a form of self-medication for dietary deficiencies (Bruinsma and Taren 1999). In other words, a constant craving for chocolate may indicate an underlying magnesium deficiency, which is best corrected with plenty of green vegetables, whole grains, and beans—and perhaps the occasional piece of very dark chocolate (70 percent cacao and above, so as to minimize the inevitable helping of sugar).

# VITAMIN K

Vitamin K is well established as being necessary for blood clotting. It also plays a crucial role in the production of proteins in the bone, and in the production of osteocalcin, which helps calcium crystallize in the bones and speeds the healing of fractures by stimulating bone growth. Interestingly, studies have found that vitamin K strengthens the bones without actually adding to their mineral density (Booth 2007). If we remember the importance of the collagen matrix for maintaining bone flexibility, this makes perfect sense.

Bear in mind that this vitamin is can be synthesized in the intestines by friendly bacteria, which can be destroyed by antibiotic use. In addition, a number of anticlotting medications such as coumadin (Warfarin), used to prevent heart attack, interfere with vitamin K production (Booth and Mayer 2000), so these drugs may contribute to osteoporosis and fractures.

Food sources are plentiful. They include lettuce, dark leafy greens, egg yolks, and fish liver oils. A paper from the Nurses' Health Study found that those who ate lettuce daily (even iceberg lettuce!) had a 45 percent lower risk of hip fracture than those who consumed lettuce less than once weekly. The amount needed daily for healthy bones is about 150 mcg per day—the amount found in 1 cup of lettuce or ½ cup of cooked kale (Feskanich et al. 1999). This is a major reason why leafy greens are such an important food for healthy bones. And it makes things very easy from a whole foods standpoint. Just have a nice salad each day and you're set!

# OTHER VITAMINS AND MINERALS

In addition to the minerals and vitamins already mentioned, nutritionist Ann Louise Gittleman, author of *Supernutrition for Menopause* (1993), points out that we also need the following nutrients to aid in bone building:

- **Boron** helps in the synthesis of estrogen and vitamin D. It is found most abundantly in dried fruits, nuts, legumes, and caviar.

- **Manganese** is essential for the utilization of vitamins B and C, the synthesis of cartilage, and bone growth and maintenance. It is found mostly in nuts, seeds, whole grains, seaweeds, and dark leafy greens.

- **Zinc** is needed for normal bone formation, as it enhances the action of vitamin D. It is found mostly in meat, eggs, seafood, oysters, pumpkin seeds, and dried beans.

- **Copper** is essential for the formation of collagen. Food sources are nuts, seeds, organ meats, and seafood.

- **Silicon** promotes the formation of bones and teeth, as well as collagen. It is found in whole grains, such as whole wheat, oats, and brown rice.

- **Vitamin B$_6$** (pyridoxine) helps strengthen collagen. The best sources are bananas, carrots, onions, sunflower seeds, and walnuts, as well as whole grains.

- **Folic acid** helps convert the amino acid homocysteine, which interferes with collagen synthesis, to the nontoxic form, cysteine. The best sources are leafy green vegetables, tuna, salmon, brown rice, beef, and beans.

If we add up all these nutrients necessary for bone health, pretty soon we'll end up with ... food!

Jokes aside, this long list of nutrients that affect bone formation may be confusing, so let's be clear about one very important fact: The process of bone remodeling (the deposition of calcium salts and the release of them back into the bloodstream to satisfy important metabolic needs) involves a system of checks and balances that keeps our metabolism in equilibrium. Directly interfering with this balance through drugs or supplementation, even when it looks like the body is doing its job incorrectly, should only be undertaken with extreme caution. I believe a better approach is to strengthen and nourish the body so it can do its own healing. This means consuming the foods that support bone health, and using the bones regularly in physical activities. Nature knows what it's doing, and we often don't. In our ignorance, we try to fix things by focusing on one side of the equation, and so risk invoking the law of unintended consequences and making things worse rather than better.

Once you realize that bones are living tissue, it becomes clear that preventing fractures is a multifaceted endeavor. Alan R. Gaby, MD, president of the American Holistic Medical Association and medical editor of the *Townsend Letter for Doctors*, points out in his book *Preventing and Reversing Osteoporosis* (1994) that to prevent fractures we need to pay attention to three factors: preventing the loss of calcium and other minerals from bone; maintaining the soft tissue components of bone, such as the proteins that give it flexibility; and making sure that the bones are capable of repairing damaged areas promptly and efficiently. That ability, of course, comes with a healthy body and strong immune system; it cannot be taken out of context.

# HEALTHY FATS

Fats have taken an incredible beating in recent years. They have practically been considered equivalent to an evil poison; numerous otherwise sane people avoid fat as if it were a direct insult to the body. So much fear and loathing are unwarranted. Fats are one of the three essential macronutrients that provide us with calories (protein and carbohydrates are the other two). As a concentrated source of energy, fat is essential in cold climates because its breakdown provides heat. A layer of fat under the skin insulates the body and helps keep it at a steady temperature, which is essential to life. This same layer of fat (perhaps a bit thicker), can produce estrogens to help women in menopause and beyond keep their hormone levels up naturally. And the kidneys, heart, liver, and other internal organs need to be surrounded by fat deposits so as to be protected and held in place.

Good-quality fats are needed for the proper function of the immune and hormonal systems; for production of bile, cholesterol, prostaglandins, and sex hormones; and for cell wall construction. They're also critical for the transport of fat-soluble vitamins such as A, D, E, and K, and therefore are closely involved in the metabolism of calcium. If we are fat-deficient, we will also be deficient in fat-soluble vitamins involved in bone metabolism, which in turn will affect our absorption of calcium (Enig 2000).

Healthy fats are high in essential fatty acids (EFAs), which are polyunsaturated and include omega-3 and omega-6, both associated with cardiovascular health, good skin and nails, lustrous hair, and a strong immune system. EFAs protect against bone loss by decreasing bone resorption (Miggiano and Gagliardi 2005). They also prevent calcium from being excreted in the urine. The best sources of EFAs are nuts, especially walnuts, seeds, and fresh fatty cold-water fish, such as salmon and mackerel.

Nature does the job right, as usual. When they are unrefined, natural fats and oils come packaged together with their natural antioxidants and other nutrients. If cows and chickens are raised on fresh grass, seeds, and no drugs, their milk, meat, and eggs have a higher proportion of monounsaturated fats and lower cholesterol.

And although saturated fats continue to be demonized, they are, in fact, necessary for many important metabolic functions (Enig and Fallon 2005):

- They constitute at least 50 percent of cell membranes.

- They help in assimilating the EFAs.

- They protect the liver from damage due to alcohol ingestion.

- They enhance the immune system.

- They have antimicrobial properties.

- And, most importantly, they play a vital role in bone modeling.

According to biochemist and nutritionist Mary Enig, Ph.D., in order for calcium deposition in the bones to be most effective, saturated fats should comprise about 50 percent of the fats in the diet (Enig and Fallon 2005). Interestingly, populations in tropical areas, where the saturated coconut and palm oils are regularly used in the diet, have very little osteoporosis. They also have very little heart disease!

Since these facts may seem somewhat surprising, let's take a look at possible explanations. Just like other tissues in the body, bones may be damaged by free radicals. These are highly reactive molecules involved in essential energy production throughout the body; they are also commonly formed by the polyunsaturated fatty acids (PUFAs). When there are too many of them, they may cause damage to tissues and cells, and contribute to cancer and heart disease. In fact, a diet high in PUFAs has been associated with bone loss (Macdonald et al. 2004). Free radicals are neutralized by antioxidant nutrients, such as vitamins C and E, carotene, and bioflavonoids. Because the tropical fats consumed in traditional societies are usually fresh and unrefined, they contain a number of additional antioxidant nutrients, such as carotene, vitamin E, and other components, which contribute to the body's nutrient stores (Enig and Fallon 2005).

These natural fats are a far cry from the bleached, refined, deodorized, hydrogenated oils and fats so widely available in our stores. I recently had the opportunity to use fresh, unrefined palm oil from Africa. It was thickish and had a deep, rich orange color. When I used it for sautéing vegetables, I needed no herbs or other seasonings because the flavor was so wonderful, close to paprika, yet without being a nightshade. The beautiful color indicated that it was full of natural carotenes and antioxidants, and thus protective against damaging free radicals and probably good for the bones. These tropical oils, when natural and unrefined, are also very resistant to becoming rancid and rarely need refrigeration.

Among the best fats to use in cooking are the following:

- Extra-virgin olive oil

- Unrefined sesame and sunflower oils

- Cold-pressed flaxseed oil (use only in unheated dishes, or add after cooking, to avoid damaging this delicate oil)

- Traditional unrefined coconut and palm oils

- Butter or cream (preferably raw) from healthy cows fed grass and raised organically

In addition, the fats in eggs and animal foods that are organically raised or wild can be consumed in their natural states as part of a wholesome eating regime. Nuts and seeds, including flaxseeds, are excellent sources the natural fats, as well as trace minerals, and have been shown to be protective of the heart as well as the immune system. Susan Lark, MD, author of the *Lark Letter*, recommends that women eat 2 to 5 tablespoons of ground flaxseed daily for the health of their bones. This provides good amounts of calcium, magnesium, and essential fatty acids, particularly the omega-3 fatty acids (Lark 2003). The latter is particularly important, as the contemporary Western diet generally provides far too high a proportion of omega-6s and few if any omega-3s.

# A Word on Cholesterol

Cholesterol is a natural substance that has a terrible reputation. This is also unwarranted. Cholesterol is classified as a lipid, although strictly speaking it's a fat-soluble steroid alcohol. There are two sources for cholesterol: *endogenous* (made by the body itself) and *exogenous* (consumed in foods). It is manufactured by the liver of all warm-blooded animals, and in humans it is a crucial component of several body structures and functions. The human liver manufactures between 800 and 1,500 mg of cholesterol daily, so the endogenous contribution to total cholesterol is considerable.

Cholesterol has many important roles in the body. One of its functions is to lubricate the blood vessels to prevent damage to their walls by the vigorously rushing bloodstream. About 90 percent of the body's total cholesterol resides in the cells, where it is a major component of cell membranes, including all of the membranes around all of the organelles inside the cells, such as the mitochondria. It maintains the right amount of both rigidity and flexibility in all of these membranes. Infants need the cholesterol in mothers' milk to help the development of their brain and eyes. In addition, it helps build hormones (including estrogen, testosterone, and the stress hormone cortisol), bile acids, and vitamin D. It also affects the bones, because cholesterol in the skin is the precursor for vitamin D manufactured by sunlight, and without that nutrient the bones cannot obtain the calcium they need.

When we eat, the fats in our meal get broken down into fatty acids, and after they pass through the intestinal wall, many of them go into the lymphatic system and straight into the blood, bypassing the liver. Why would they do such a thing? Everything else we eat goes to the liver first, but not the fats. The fats are transported in large particles called chylomicrons, which are carried all around the body by the blood and act like delivery trucks, dropping off lipids at all the cells that require them. There they provide energy, insulate against temperature extremes, protect against shock, maintain the cell membranes, and build various compounds, such as hormones. As they drop off their cargo, the chylomicrons get smaller and smaller, and after fourteen hours only a few bits and pieces remain, which are picked up by the liver and recycled.

Meanwhile, the liver makes cholesterol, triglycerides, and other fatty acids, and packages them with proteins as very low-density lipoproteins (VLDLs), which are also sent out as delivery trucks with the materials that the cells need. As the VLDLs lose triglycerides, they become the more familiar low-density lipoprotein (LDL or "bad" cholesterol), which is proportionately higher in cholesterol. The LDLs keep traveling around, bringing their content to the heart muscle, the fat stores, the mammary glands, the endocrine glands, and other sites, which use these lipids to build or repair their membranes, make hormones, or store them for energy and later use. Our smart liver then makes high-density lipoprotein (HDL, or "good" cholesterol), which acts as a cleaning crew. It's sent out to pick up unused cholesterol from the cells and transport them back to the liver for cleanup or recycling (Whitney and Rolfes 2005).

It should now be obvious that cholesterol is an essential substance for proper physical functioning. There is no such thing as "bad" or "good" cholesterol; there are just aspects of cholesterol with different functions. When more cholesterol is consumed, less is made by the liver. Conversely, when less is consumed, more is made in the body. Not only that, the more cholesterol consumed, the less absorbed. This is why a high-protein diet can actually cause a person's cholesterol levels to go down. On the other hand, those who go on a low-fat, high-carbohydrate diet find their LDL and triglycerides going up and their HDL going down, the opposite of the ideal according to conventional medical wisdom. But the body's wisdom is not to be dismissed; this reaction could mean that there isn't enough cholesterol for the body's needs, so the body is conserving what it has.

There is controversy about the dangers of cholesterol. The International Network of Cholesterol Skeptics is a coalition of scientists who disagree with the theory that cholesterol causes heart disease (www.thincs.org). In his book *The Cholesterol Myths: Exposing the Fallacy That Saturated Fat and Cholesterol Cause Heart Disease* (2000), Swedish physician and researcher Uffe Ravnskov charges that the majority of the review studies that support a connection between cholesterol and heart disease are seriously biased, that they ignore data that contradict the theory, and that they are written by researchers who get their major funding from pharmaceutical companies that make anticholesterol drugs, which are among the top-selling medications. In fact, populations that consume diets high in natural saturated fats have little or no heart disease. For example, a study of residents of two Polynesian atolls showed that the high consumption of coconut oil, while associated with higher cholesterol levels, is associated with a low incidence of cardiovascular heart disease (Prior et al. 1981).

That said, if high cholesterol of any variety is present *with other symptoms of ill health*, lifestyle changes are in order to reduce the risk of disease. Here are some specific recommendations:

- Substantially increase your intake of fresh vegetables, salads, fruits, whole grains, and beans.

- Lower or eliminate consumption of all kinds of added sugars and refined grain products.

- Keep your weight within a healthy range.

- Get a reasonable amount of regular physical activity every day.

- Attend to your emotional health and well-being.

All of these strategies will contribute to better health and the reduction of heart disease risk. They will also contribute to healthier bones!

## Unhealthy Fats

As nutritionist Udo Erasmus said so cogently, some fats heal, and some fats kill (1993). The unhealthy fats are those that are refined, heated, or hydrogenated. They are found in fried foods, commercially processed products, and animals raised on poor diets, drugs, and no exercise. Here are specific fats to avoid:

- Refined, bleached, and deodorized oils, including corn, safflower, soy, and canola, all fats with no taste (an indication that they contain no trace nutrients)

- Hydrogenated and partially hydrogenated fats such as margarine and shortening, because they're high in trans-fatty acids, which have been implicated in a wide variety of health problems

- Any fat heated above the temperature of boiling water, or about 200°F

- Fats from animals raised by conventional, agribusiness methods

- Pasteurized whole milk, butter, cream, yogurt, ice cream, and cheese from commercially raised cows, given antibiotics, hormones, and the equivalent of junk food instead of their natural diet of plain grass and water

Among the worst sources of fats are chips and snacks, crisp baked goods (crispness is always a sign of high saturated fat content, often in the form of hydrogenated margarine or shortenings), candies, and commercial milk products, especially commercial ice cream (because of its high content of partially hydrogenated fats). Trans fats created by the hydrogenation process are at the top of the list of fats to avoid, as they contribute to cardiovascular disease, infertility, immune system dysfunction, cancer, and osteoporosis (Shikany and White 2000; Zaloga et al. 2006). And because they slow down the digestive process by cutting down the secretion of hydrochloric acid in the stomach, these fats also contribute to slow digestion, indigestion, and poor absorption of nutrients.

On a standard American diet of processed and fast foods, it is entirely possible to consume 40 percent or more of calories from unhealthy fats and trans fats, such as partially hydrogenated vegetable oils. This diet, low in vegetables and high in protein, refined carbohydrates, and unhealthy fats, creates an increased tendency toward an acidic condition in the body, which in turn removes calcium from the bones, particularly when accompanied by the regular consumption of soft drinks and sweets. I will discuss this further in the section on the acid-alkaline balance in the next chapter.

# STRAIN, STRESS, AND MOVEMENT

Now here is some information that probably won't come as news to you: Exercise is good for the skeleton. Movement and weight-bearing exercise put stress on the long bones of the arms and legs, a factor essential to the continued process of bone deposition. When movement is lacking, as with sedentary or bedridden people, bones invariably lose mass. The influence of gravity is crucial. Astronauts in space lost bone mass during weightlessness until they began doing special exercises to prevent this problem, stressing their muscles and bones against fixed points in the spacecraft cabin.

The body needs to move. The way it is designed, walking is the movement that most efficiently puts just enough gentle strain on the bones to promote their continued remodeling. It also doesn't cost anything, and so it is the easiest and most natural way to ensure continued bone health. Brisk walking or race walking provide additional benefits. In fact, an article in *New York Magazine* attributes the longer life of New York City residents to the fact that they walk a lot and do so at a fast clip (Thompson 2007). Jogging and running, if the knees allow it, are also beneficial, but not essential. Golfing, as long as it involves walking and not riding in a cart, is an excellent if high-priced way to protect your bones.

How does this work? When the heel hits the ground while walking, vibrations travel the length of the leg bones, and the stress creates a piezoelectric effect all along them, keeping the bone crystals together as well as attracting calcium from the blood and encouraging it to be deposited onto the bone. Walking briskly on firm ground either barefoot or in shoes *with thin soles* is one simple way to encourage this process, and is in fact how human beings have been doing it for thousands of years. So what about those very thick rubber-soled sneakers? Perhaps thin-soled tennis shoes or light moccasins might be better for bone deposition.

There are other downsides to thick rubber soles. An article in the *Tufts University Health and Nutrition Letter* pointed out that athletic shoes with thick, spongy soles are the worst kind for maintaining balance and might lead to falls, especially in older people, because they don't allow for an accurate perception of where your feet are in relation to the ground (Tufts University 1997). A simple way to handle this issue is to always walk barefoot around the house; that way all of the twenty-seven bones in each foot get a good deal of exercise.

In addition, by improving posture and balance, all forms of exercise can lower the risk of falls, which may result in fractures. Not only that, a 1997 study by Dr. Laurence Kushi of the University of Minnesota School of Public Health in Minneapolis found that postmenopausal women who engaged in moderate activity (bowling, gardening, or long walks) four or more times weekly were 33 percent less likely to die during the study than sedentary women (Kushi et al. 1997).

It is really important for young women to do regular physical exercise and lift some type of weight so as to build good bone mass early in life. However, if you're older, don't fret; bone mass can be increased at any age with exercise. One study in a nursing home had sedentary older women start an exercise program by lifting soup cans—imagine muscles so weak from disuse that soup cans are heavy! The women experienced significant increases in strength and mobility, something worth keeping in mind when you hear that bone mass peaks at age thirty and it's only downhill from there (Evans 1995, 1999).

All this is no news to you, I'm sure; however, a little reminder is always good. And no, there are no exercise pills. You have to do it yourself. See chapter 7 for specific recommendations on exercise.

# HORMONAL INFLUENCES

A number of hormones regulate the health of our bones, including calcium-regulating hormones, sex hormones, and others.

## Calcium-Regulating Hormones

Two hormones regulate the movement of calcium into and out of bone. The first is calcitonin, secreted by the thyroid gland, located below the Adam's apple, in response to high amounts of calcium in the blood; this hormone lowers blood calcium by preventing bone resorption. The other hormone is parathyroid hormone, now sometimes called parathormone, secreted by the four parathyroid glands, located on the four corners of the thyroid. The release of this hormone, triggered by below-normal levels of calcium in the blood, encourages bone resorption so as to raise those levels once again.

## Sex Hormones

Estrogen and testosterone both promote the deposition of bone. For women of menopausal age and older, diminished production of estrogen promotes bone loss through lack of rebuilding. In other words, bone resorption continues in order to satisfy the needs of the blood, muscles, heart, and nervous system for calcium and other minerals, but because deposition is reduced, bone density decreases. Age-related diminishment of androgens in men has also been shown to cause bone loss via the same process. I'll discuss estrogen replacement therapy more fully in chapter 4.

## Other Systemic Hormones

The human endocrine system is incredibly complex and delicately balanced. The hormones it secretes are speedy messengers carrying very precise information. It's not unlike an internal Internet that brings communication from one end of the body to the other at amazing speeds. Hundreds of different hormones affect every system in the body, and all of these systems rely on accurate communication. While many hormones can influence bone metabolism, here are four of the most noteworthy:

- **Growth hormone**, secreted by the pituitary gland, is essential for growth in general, and especially for the growth of the skeleton at puberty. It may stimulate both osteoclasts and osteoblasts, but it's more dominant on the bone formation process while the body grows.

- **Thyroid hormones** influence the energy production of all cells and stimulate bone turnover. Deficiency of these hormones can cause too much bone breakdown and thus contribute to weaker bones.

- **Cortisol**, secreted by the adrenal glands (located on top of the kidneys), regulates metabolism and the response to injury and stress. The "three bears rule" applies to cortisol: Too little is detrimental to bone development, and too much blocks bone growth. Most importantly, synthetic forms of this hormone (the steroids and glucocorticoids used in many pharmacological drugs), can cause severe and sometimes rapid bone loss.

- **Insulin**, produced by the pancreas, also affects the skeleton. A deficiency of this hormone can impair the body's response to signals for bone growth.

# WATER

Although we think of water as a soft, fluid substance, it can, in fact, be considered the strongest substance on earth. Think of it this way: Water can break rocks and glass, lift enormous weight in hydraulic lifts, and ravage everything in its path during a flood. It is also the basis of all life on this planet.

Our human bodies are 60 to 70 percent water by weight. This water is within and around our cells, in our secretions, our blood, and our tissues. It travels freely throughout the body, passing through membranes and organs with equal ease. Our bones contain about 25 percent water by weight (American Society for Bone and Mineral Research 2004), and this water is essential for keeping them structurally strong, much as the sap in a tree keeps it from breaking. Dry trees will crack and splinter, and dry bones may do the same. In fact, studies with nuclear resonance imaging have found that very thin layers of water between the collagen fibers and the bone mineral matter may be an important element in the stability of bone matter (Wilson et al. 2005).

An interesting thing that happened to me in this respect is the story of my nails, which, like bones, need good minerals for proper growth. For years and years I had very thin, soft nails that peeled into layers and tore very easily. There were times, usually during the summer, when my nails seemed to strengthen, but then they would weaken again. I tried a variety of dietary approaches and even asked several doctors and nutritionists, but nothing worked. Finally, only about a year before writing this book, I got really fed up and decided to engage in a serious regime of nutritional supplements for my nails. I almost never use supplements because I feel they unbalance the body, but I thought maybe this was the time. So I bought three or four different products, some recommended by a new doctor I had consulted, and got ready to embark on this new adventure. However, I kept forgetting about it. Then one day I was looking at my nails and deciding yet again to get into my new regime, when I got the very strong intuitive feeling that I was *dry*. My nails were breaking because they were dry. I resolved to make sure I drank eight glasses of water—plain spring water—per day (instead of my usual three or four), and kept to the regime. Within a week I could tell my nails were stronger, and within a month I had good, normal, strong nails that no longer peeled or broke. I returned all of the unopened supplements to my natural food store. At this time, about a year later, I have nice strong nails the way I always wanted. The only thing I regret is that it took me more than twenty years to figure this out. So if you have a similar problem, I hope I'm saving you some time.

According to Fereydoon Batmanghelidj, MD, author of *Your Body's Many Cries for Water* (1995), we may ignore, not recognize, or lose our sense of thirst, and thereby become mildly or chronically dehydrated. Among the symptoms of such dehydration are asthma, high blood pressure, diabetes, and pain in general, including stomach, angina, and joint pain, as well as low back pain, one of the indicators of possible osteoporosis. A sufficient intake of clean water is essential for the proper function of the entire body as well as the strength of the bones. About eight or ten glasses daily is the ideal.

Based on earlier studies I had undertaken, for a long time I disagreed with this viewpoint. Specifically, I thought that when we eat more whole grains, beans, and vegetables, we need less water because there is so much water in the cooked grains and beans, and of course in the vegetables as well. Therefore, drinking much more than what one needs might overwork the kidneys. But as time went on I realized that, once again, context counts, and I had to broaden my viewpoint. The amount of water you need depends on whatever else there is in your diet. In other words, the more dry or low-water foods you eat, the more water you need.

Dry or low-water foods include animal protein, baked flour products of any kind, nuts, seeds, and sweets. High-water products include fresh vegetables, fruits, and cooked whole grains and beans. Salty liquids, caffeine, alcohol, and sweetened drinks don't count as water because they are actually diuretics. Another part of this picture is how often during the day you eat. If you eat just two or three meals a day with no snacks, you need to drink some water every hour or so, and if you snack on dry foods, like nuts or dried fruits or snack bars, you absolutely must take in some water with them.

In addition, water requirements vary according to other factors, such as activity level and climate. An acquaintance from Japan told me that dogs and cats in that country hardly ever drink because of the constant humidity in the air of that island nation.

How do we know if we've had enough water? Back to the "three bears rule": Enough means not too much or too little; it should be just right. If you are well hydrated, your urine will be pale (unless you've taken B vitamins) and abundant, and you won't have to empty your bladder more often than every three hours or so. If the need to urinate is more frequent, there could be either too much water intake or some organic disorder, such as kidney trouble or diabetes. An excess of water consumption, which may be common with athletes who sweat heavily or even people on weight-loss diets, can lower the relative concentration of minerals (electrolytes) in the blood, especially sodium, which can cause a condition called hyponatremia, or too little sodium in the blood. Symptoms include severe headache, vomiting, puffiness from water retention, confusion, cramps, and even seizures. Athletes and people who sweat more than is common shouldn't restrict their salt intake and should consume salty snacks, such as salty pretzels or chips, olives, or anchovies, anytime they sweat heavily. They should also consult with their trainer, health care professional, or another reliable source to learn more about how best to maintain good hydration and electrolyte balance.

If your urine is dark and scant and you don't have to void your bladder often, you aren't drinking enough water. Sometimes when people don't drink enough water during the day, they don't urinate much, yet they need to get up during the night to do so. In these cases, drinking more during the day is the answer, so as to stimulate the kidneys to do their job during the daylight hours. Symptoms of more serious dehydration include headache, nausea, dizziness, lack of focus or clumsiness, lack of sweat in the heat, and confusion. Some of these symptoms are similar to those of hyponatremia, but a few appropriate questions, as well as the observation of whether one is sweating or not, should help determine the problem.

I find that room temperature water is best, rather than ice-cold, because it's easier for the body to accept and assimilate rapidly. Normal body temperature is 98.6°F, so bringing 40°F water up to that level takes the body a lot more time and energy than dealing with 70°F water. To add some electrolytes, a pinch of good sea salt in a glass of water is a good idea.

What kind of water should we be drinking? What about tap water? Unfortunately, while tap water can be considered reasonably clean, in most communities it has had various chemicals added, such as chlorine and fluoride. It's easy enough to eliminate the chlorine; simply draw the water and then let it sit uncovered for a couple of hours so the chlorine can evaporate. Fluoride, on the other hand, won't evaporate. You may be under the impression that it's a benign or even beneficial substance that helps prevent cavities, but the truth is it's closer to a medication that we're forced to consume in most municipal water supplies. (More on fluoride in the next chapter.) Avoid fluoridated water at all costs.

To obtain the cleanest water possible, either use a good filter or purchase good-quality spring water in bottles—or, if you're lucky enough, use fresh water from your own brook, spring, or well. There are many types of water filters on the market, and certainly one for every budget. There are filters in a pitcher that you can keep in the refrigerator or on the countertop, and others that are hooked up to the faucet, to the water supply under the sink, or even to the water supply of the whole house. Because most filters don't remove fluoride, ask specifically about this issue before you purchase a filter. If you have your own water source, make sure to have the water tested for impurities, bacteria, and parasites from time to time. I don't recommend distilled water because it has been stripped of its beneficial minerals. It is quite akin to white sugar in that regard, and I maintain that it draws minerals out of the body, and the bones, simply by osmotic pressure. Good water should nourish plants and support fish; if it doesn't, it's lacking something.

So make sure your water supply is the best you can get. If you aren't totally sure about it, or if you find yourself having to drink water you didn't choose or filter yourself, do something very simple: Thank the water for being there and quenching your thirst. That way you at least put some good thought and energy into what you're drinking; it won't hurt, and it may even help.

# THE ROLE OF SODIUM

Sodium has an undeservedly bad reputation. This is unfortunate, as it is absolutely crucial to our health. It is an alkalizing mineral that is found abundantly in our bodies, especially in the fluids both outside and within all our cells, as well as in the bones. It works with potassium to balance the acid-alkaline factors in the bloodstream, and helps regulate water balance, muscle contraction, and nerve stimulation. It is essential for the proper function of our cells, nerves, and metabolism. Sodium also helps keep the other essential minerals dissolved in our blood, and so avoids the buildup of deposits. It aids in purging carbon dioxide (which we breathe out) from the body and stimulates the production of hydrochloric acid in the stomach, thereby assisting digestion.

Sodium is found abundantly in nature and throughout our food supply, and not just in the form of sodium chloride, as in table salt. It's in all natural foods, such as meat, beans, and vegetables, in easily absorbable form. This isn't really a problem. Where we may run into trouble is with excessive added salt, as well as the sodium found in many sodium-based ingredients, additives, and preservatives in commercial foods. Baked goods that contain baking soda (bicarbonate of sodium) and baking powder (which contains baking soda) can be a highly significant, though often over-looked, source of sodium. Any ingredient with the word "sodium" or "soda" in it contains sodium salts. A quick look at a packaged food's ingredient list will tell you if there is sodium in it; the nutrition label will say how much. Here are some additives to watch for in ingredient lists:

- Monosodium glutamate

- Sodium benzoate

- Sodium bisulfite

- Sodium caseinate

- Sodium citrate

- Sodium nitrite

- Sodium propionate

- Sodium stearoyl lactylate

The average appropriate sodium intake has been estimated by the National Research Council to be 2,300 mg per day, the amount in about 1 teaspoon of salt (Institute of Medicine 2004). While it is a necessary and essential mineral, a number of studies have shown that sodium will increase the urinary excretion of calcium, indicating bone loss, when consumed in excess (more than 3,000 mg per day). However, a more recent study, published in the journal *Food and Chemical Toxicology*, indicates that higher calcium loss through the urine in response to salt intake only occurs in a minority of humans (Cohen and Roe 2000).

In addition, a sixteen-year study at the UCLA School of Medicine found that the effects of sodium intake on bone mineral density were not significant, except that for *men*, increased sodium intake actually increased bone mineral density in the arm bones (Greendale et al. 1994). On the other hand, a 1995 study on postmenopausal women at the University of Western Australia found that a reduction in bone loss equivalent to a daily dietary *increase* of about 900 mg of calcium can be achieved by simply reducing intake of sodium to about 1,200 mg per day (Devine et al. 1995). And to further underscore how interrelated mineral levels in the body are, a study at the Department of Food and Nutritional Sciences at the University College of Cork, Ireland, found that increased potassium intake may neutralize the effects of sodium (Harrington and Cashman 2003).

So here is the upshot: Modest amounts of salt in the diet will not damage the bones, particularly if it's sea salt, which has additional trace minerals—between 4 and 10 percent; therefore, the sodium chloride content may be as low as 90 percent, compared to 98 percent for commercial table salt. Commercial foods with a high sodium content from additives may damage the bones, while potassium intake will counteract the sodium and thereby protect the bones. In other words, back to the vegetables, the best sources of potassium!

If you choose to use salt, the best kind is unrefined, natural salt from clean ocean waters or clean inland salt mines (the remnants of ancient oceans). There are considerable differences between the traditional salt obtained from evaporation of seawater (known as sea salt), that mined from salt mines, and the pure, white, free-flowing substance most common at the supermarket. Commercial table salt contains a number of sodium-based additives, such as sodium silicoaluminate and yellow prussiate of soda, plus potassium iodide and additional additives of high cosmetic value but questionable in terms of health.

Although it can be somewhat expensive, fleur du sel ("flower of salt" in French) is a good choice for adding sparingly at the table. Gray sea salt is the best type to use in cooking, in modest amounts measured in sprinkles. The food should never taste salty; use just enough salt to brighten all of the other flavors in the food.

Our concern about excess sodium in the diet should be reserved mostly for processed foods. Many of the studies on salt and calcium were done with rats, and that information is not always applicable to humans. The sodium in natural foods, such as meat or celery, is balanced by the presence of other minerals, so these are beneficial sources that give us the sodium we need in a balanced way and pose no problem.

Bones are complex structures. They rely on a variety of factors, all working together, in order to be healthy. Single nutrients in pill form may not cover all the requirements (especially exercise!). By the same token, there are may ways in which bones can be weakened, and it's important that we know what they are so we can avoid them. The next chapter takes a close look at this issue.

# CHAPTER 4

# What Weakens Our Bones? It's More Than Menopause

*My bones consumed away through my daily complaining.*

—Psalms 32:3

What weakens our bones is, of course, the crux of the matter. How can we know what we should be doing about bone thinning and fragility if we don't know what caused the problem in the first place? We saw that bone health is a very complex system, making it obvious that the weakening of bones can be caused by many factors. Wouldn't it be a waste of time and money to take calcium pills when what the body needs is magnesium? There are many aspects of our contemporary lifestyle that contribute to osteoporosis.

When they contain insufficient calcium salts, the bones become porous and soft; with insufficient protein or collagen, they become brittle. Osteoporosis involves a decrease in both protein and calcium, due to faulty remodeling (more being taken out than is put in), so the bones become both porous *and* brittle. This lack of bone deposition could be caused by a low supply of the necessary nutrients, such as calcium or protein. However, a lack of nutrients is not the only cause. The highest incidence of osteoporosis is found in the United States and Scandinavia, countries that consume an abundance of milk products, which are high in both protein and calcium (Sanson 2003). Something else must be at work here. It could be that the nutrients aren't absorbed, or they could be drained or counteracted by other elements.

Before we take a closer look at those possibilities, let's briefly consider the role of menopause, since it receives so much attention. Over and over again, women hear that once they grow older and their ovaries are producing less estrogen, bone loss inevitably follows and it's time for medication. I consider this a foolish notion. To make the point better than I can, let me quote Professor John A. Kanis, from the World Health Organization Collaborating Centre for Metabolic Bone Diseases at the University of Sheffield Medical School in Great Britain. He writes in the journal *Bone*, "The importance of the menopause to the problems of osteoporosis has been overemphasized." Other factors, he says, are involved in the increase in hip fracture risk that has occurred in many countries. The causes clearly aren't related to menopause only, "because these phenomena are observed in both men and women" (Kanis 1996, 185S).

In other words, even though osteoporosis and bone fractures occur during the later stages of a woman's life, menopause isn't the *cause* of these problems. They are only temporally related. More important for bone health is how we use our bodies, and especially what we eat.

## A LACK OR A DRAIN?

What we eat both builds and fuels every part of our bodies. Even though we have the notion that our bones just "sit there" and do nothing, the foods we consume affect them both directly and indirectly: directly, because if we don't consume enough vitamin D, calcium, and protein, they will be unable to rebuild themselves; and indirectly, because as so many of the nutrients interrelate, a deficiency of one (vitamin D, for example) can cause a deficiency in another (calcium), even if there is a sufficient quantity of the second in the diet. In addition, there are aspects of our diet that impact our bones because they cause an active nutrient loss, or drain; over time, this drain can cause as much trouble as any overt deficiency. One important concept that will help us understand the role and interrelationship of calcium and other minerals much more clearly is the acid-alkaline balance. Let's take a look at this important but little-understood dynamic.

### Acid-Alkaline Balance

The acid-alkaline (or acid-base) balance is expressed in terms of the pH (or power of hydrogen) scale, which ranges from 0 to 14. A pH of 7 is neutral, below 7 is acid, and above 7 is alkaline. *Acids* are substances with missing electrons, so their tendency is to go steal electrons elsewhere, and that thieving tendency makes them corrosive. In the body, acids generally result from metabolic processes such as moving or breathing; these acids are then either excreted or *buffered* (neutralized) by minerals or mineral salts, which in turn are considered *alkaline* (or basic). For the proper function of our metabolism, our blood plasma has to be slightly alkaline, at a pH of about 7.45. This is a highly delicate balance, and going off even a little on either side can have serious consequences, including death: For example, an alkaline blood plasma pH of 7.9 may precipitate lockjaw or tetany and be fatal, while an acid pH of 6.9 brings about diabetic coma and may also be fatal. With a correct blood pH, the body is in *homeostasis*, or inner balance. It's important to remember that minerals buffer acids.

In yet another case of the "three bears rule," the body has a number of mechanisms to keep the acid-alkaline balance just right:

- In the process of breathing, the cells exhale carbonic acid, which becomes carbon dioxide and is expelled through the lungs, lowering the body's acid load.

- The movement of muscles creates lactic acid due to the breakdown of glycogen (stored carbohydrate) to produce energy, increasing acidity.

- The kidneys regulate the acid-alkaline balance in the blood by excreting urine that is more acid or more alkaline according to what needs to be eliminated.

- If the blood becomes too acid, the bones release calcium and other buffering minerals into the bloodstream through resorption to rebalance the pH.

- The foods we eat contribute to either an acid or an alkaline environment *once they're metabolized*. Their effect depends on the residue they leave behind: If they leave acids (carbonic, phosphoric, or sulfuric) they are *acid-forming*. If they leave buffering minerals (mostly calcium, iron, magnesium, potassium, and sodium), they are *alkalizing*.

Here's a simple concept to help you remember this model: The more minerals there are in a food, the more it alkalizes the body. Most produce is alkalizing because it leaves behind an alkaline residue in the form of the minerals mentioned above. Alkalizing foods include fruits, vegetables, seaweeds, soy sauce, miso, and salt. Protein and carbohydrate foods are acid-forming because they leave behind an acid residue; acid-forming foods include sugar, flour, beans, grains, fish, poultry, meat, and eggs (Colbin 1999).

A slight tilt toward acidity in the bloodstream, called *acidosis* (or, if you will, a reduction of alkalinity), can remove calcium from the bones so as to alkalize the blood (Ott 2004). Studies done on mice at the University of Rochester School of Medicine and Dentistry have shown that calcium does indeed leave the bones when they are in an acid environment. In other words, metabolic acidosis stimulates bone resorption and inhibits bone formation (Krieger, Frick, and Bushinsky 2004).

Dr. T. Colin Campbell of Cornell University, in collaboration with Oxford University and the Institute of Nutrition and Food Hygiene of the Chinese Academy of Preventive Medicine in Beijing, conducted a famous study of the dietary patterns and nutritional status of Chinese people in the early 1990s. That study showed clearly that the levels of acids and calcium in the urine of middle-aged and elderly women was influenced considerably by their diet. The consumption of acid-forming foods increased calcium excretion in the urine. Animal protein appeared to be one of the culprits, whereas plant protein intake wasn't related to urinary calcium excretion (Campbell and Campbell 2005). This finding may be one of the reasons why some studies show that vegetarians have less osteoporosis than meat eaters.

So, metabolic acidosis from excessive consumption of acid-forming foods generally has a *calcium-wasting* effect, draining calcium and other minerals from the bones. Eating meat is just one possible cause of acidosis. More commonly it's due to over-consumption of flour or sugar, both of which are acid-forming. Therefore, if people eat a lot of refined carbohydrates, the major influences weakening bone health would be the pasta, cookies, cakes, muffins, white breads, and white rice so ubiquitous in our modern food supply. In addition, we are emerging from a long spell of low-fat eating, which encouraged many people to load up on carbs without regard to whether they were based on whole grains or laden with refined sugar. While much attention has been paid to protein in regard to bone loss, refined carbohydrates have received relatively little notice, mostly because of the unfortunate misconception that "all carbohydrates are equal." However, they clearly are not the same, as anyone who's tasted the difference between whole grain bread and white bread can tell you. Christiane Northrup, MD, author of *The Wisdom of Menopause* (2006), pointed out to me that osteoporosis occurs most frequently in countries where the diet includes the habitual use of refined carbohydrate foods (personal communication).

Here's a list of foods that leave behind acids (acid-forming), those that are buffers, and those that leave bases (alkalizing) once they are metabolized:

## ACID-FORMING FOODS

- Alcohol
- Sugar
- Oils
- Nuts
- Seeds
- Flour

- Whole grains
- Beans
- Fish
- Poultry
- Meat
- Eggs

## BUFFERS

- Yogurt

- Milk

- Cheese

- Tofu (if made with calcium carbonate)

## ALKALIZING FOODS

- Juices

- Fruit

- Green vegetables

- Green beans

- Potatoes (because they contain solanine, an alkaloid)

- Seaweeds (sea vegetables)

- Soy sauce

- Miso

- Salt

Milk products and tofu (if made with calcium carbonate) are buffer foods; they will balance either side because they contain both calcium (which is alkalizing) and protein (which is acid-forming). Thus, if a diet is high in sugar, flour, or meat and low in vegetables and fruit, dairy products will help alkalize the body because of their calcium content. Conversely, if a diet is high in alkalizing fruits, green vegetables, and potatoes and low in protein or grains, dairy products will provide supplementary acid-forming protein.

The trick, of course, is to eat from both the acid-forming and the alkalizing groups. The body demands balance. Eating too high a proportion of acid-forming foods will draw minerals out of the teeth and bones, whereas eating a high proportion of alkalizing foods often tends to create cravings for sweets or carbohydrates, as many vegetarians will attest to, in order to bring in some counterbalancing acid-forming foods.

The best alkalizing foods, especially in a diet with few or no milk products, as I recommend, are plenty of leafy green vegetables, cooked or raw (kale, collard greens, mustard greens, watercress, arugula, and so on); roots (such as carrots, turnips, parsnips, and radishes); broccoli; squashes; and especially chopped fresh parsley (as raw parsley in its whole form is tough and bitter, it is classically used chopped.) Parsley contains both calcium and vitamin C, as well as ergosterol, a precursor of vitamin D, which helps the body absorb and utilize the calcium. I am not keen on recommending spinach and chard. Even though they are rich in calcium, they are also high in oxalic acid, which interferes with the absorption of calcium.

# FACTORS THAT DEPLETE CALCIUM AND OTHER MINERALS

We know that a lack of "income" will lower our bone "assets"; but too many "expenses," using up what comes in and more, will do the same. Therefore, let's take a close look at the many different dietary and lifestyle factors that can lead to unhealthy amounts of withdrawal of minerals from our bones.

## Acid-Forming Foods

As we've seen, acid-forming foods promote a tendency toward acidosis in the bloodstream; to counteract this, calcium and other minerals are withdrawn from the bones. In other words, bone resorption increases to rebalance the blood, and then the calcium and other minerals are excreted in the urine. Increased consumption of alkalizing foods can balance this equation by replacing the minerals borrowed from the bones. On the other hand, if the diet is low in alkalizing vegetables and other mineral-rich foods and this persists year after year, the calcium and other minerals needed for bone deposition would remain insufficient and the "expenses" of bone resorption would exceed the "income."

To be perfectly clear: Because their metabolic by-products include carbonic acid, carbohydrate foods are seriously acid-forming. And while whole grains at least have some beneficial fiber, trace minerals, and vitamin E in them, refined grains and flours, stripped of their bran and germ, are missing these natural nutrients. This makes them more acidifying. The same is true of the sugar removed from sugarcane and sugar beets. While the original source has plenty of water, fiber, and minerals, the refined crystallized carbohydrate we put in coffee and pastries has none left; it is 99 percent pure carbohydrate. Thus, regular consumption of white flour, white rice, and refined sugar—as well as high-fructose corn syrup—will contribute mightily to bone weakness. These are, without a doubt in my mind, the worst bone-damaging foods. Perhaps that explains the high rates of osteoporosis in Western countries, where most people regularly consume a high proportion of white bread, pasta, sugared breakfast cereals, sweet snacks, and pastries. There's even sugar in our toothpaste!

## Vegetarian or Not?

Since the early 1980s, when the concern with bone health began, many people have focused on the excess of animal proteins in the diet and found them damaging. A number of studies determined that the acid residue of protein foods is bad for the bones. However, it turns out that meat itself is not the culprit. In fact, the theory that animal proteins such as red meat cause bone loss was debunked as early as the 1980s by the studies of Herta Spencer, of the Veterans Administration Hospital in Hines, Illinois. Dr. Spencer found that studies correlating calcium loss with high-protein diets used highly processed isolated amino acids from milk or eggs. It turns out that complex dietary proteins from whole food sources, including red meat, don't cause calcium loss (Spencer and Kramer 1987).

The observations of Weston Price, DDS, author of *Nutrition and Physical Degeneration* (1979), bear out that view. Dr. Price traveled all over the world in the early 1930s, studying the health, dental health, and diet of traditional societies. Like other anthropologists before and after him, he found no people subsisting on only plant foods, although these do comprise a considerable percentage of native diets. He also found that traditional people often go to great trouble to obtain nutrient-rich fish, eggs, and other animal foods for pregnant women and those getting ready for parenthood. Dr. Price's book clearly demonstrates that traditional cultures with diets high in fish and meat have excellent bone health, as long as they also consume plenty of animal fats and vegetables.

The healthiest people he found in terms of bones and teeth were six tribes in sub-Saharan Africa that subsisted mostly on the meat, milk, and blood of cows. These six cattle-herding tribes were completely free of cavities and had strong, straight teeth and bones. Agricultural tribes, on the other hand, such as the Kikuyu and Wakamba, who consumed sweet potatoes, corn, beans, millet, and sorghum, plus small animals and insects, had decay in 5 to 6 percent of all teeth (in the United States as many as 75 percent of all teeth have decay). According to the *Price-Pottenger Nutrition Foundation Health Journal*, one of the healthiest tribes that Dr. Price found, the Sudanese Dinkas, lived on a diet consisting mainly of fish and cereal grains (Fallon and Enig 1999).

On the other hand, Dr. Price found countless cases of dental and skeletal defects (including caries, bone and jaw malformations, and clubfoot) among traditional peoples who had switched to the "civilized" diet of white bread, sugar, jam, sweetened condensed milk, canned vegetables, and alcohol. The natives who remained on their traditional diet were, on the other hand, found to be without these defects and in good health, regardless of the amount of protein consumed (Price 1979).

Clearly, it is not necessary to be vegetarian in order to have healthy bones. It also isn't necessary to eat meat. What *is* necessary is to eat lots of vegetables of many colors, enough protein, and enough good-quality fats. If you doubt that vegetables can provide sufficient nutrients for bone health, bear in mind that, in their natural state, the animals with the biggest bones (such as elephants, giraffes, cows, and horses) all primarily subsist on leafy greens.

# Cane Sugar and Other Refined Sweeteners

More than forty years ago I noticed that eating foods with added sugar made me extremely tired in the mornings. If a restaurant put a little sugar in the water to boil carrots, I would get "sugar eyes"—my term for a sense of glued eyes in the morning as I tried to wake up. I was habitually late for work, where I tried to get alert with a cup of coffee and a doughnut like everyone else seemed to do. I didn't realize sugar was the culprit until I stopped putting sugar in my coffee and replaced doughnuts with hot unsweetened cereal. After three days of this new regime, I got up early and had clear eyes—not "sugar eyes." I was alert and awake. What a discovery!

Feeling well is a great incentive. After that experience I pretty much cut out refined sugar from my diet. Every so often I'd stray, but the fatigue and "sugar eyes" always put me back on track. I also noticed that my moods changed dramatically once I quit eating sugar. From my usual slight malaise, a vague sensation of blues or minor depression, I went to feeling emotionally even and then really good most of the time. What surprised me was that such experiences were dismissed by mainstream nutritionists, and that other parents were horrified when I mentioned that I gave my children no cookies, ice cream, or candy with added sugar—*ever*. That was because early on I found, as do many parents, that kids often go crazy when they eat too much sugar.

So what is this substance that we are so enthralled with? Or, should I say, that we're so addicted to? Crystalline white cane sugar is refined from sugarcane by crushing the cane, processing the juice and evaporating it, then bleaching and deodorizing the resulting crystals until they are pure white. (A similar process is used to make sugar from sugar beets.) It takes about 17 feet of sugarcane to come up with 1 cup of white sugar. I know this because I once called a sugar factory and we worked out the numbers. If you visualize this relationship—17 feet to 1 cup—you realize that the refined cane sugar has a lot missing that is present in the original: It has none of the vitamins and minerals found in the plant, let alone any of the protein and fiber. This lack is registered by the body and creates an imbalance, or what could be called a "nutritional debt" of the missing nutrients, such as fiber, vitamin D, calcium, and iron.

It is also missing the water, so consuming sugar will make you actually thirsty. A 20-ounce can of cola may have as much as 15 teaspoons of sugar, so it can actually keep you thirsty, with the end result that you keep drinking it. A quick test will show you how insidious our thirst for soda is. To see how it really tastes and whether it actually quenches your thirst, try drinking some room-temperature cola, and note both the taste and how it makes you feel. You'll probably wonder how people can bear to drink this stuff all the time. They are tricked into continued consumption because these drinks are served ice-cold, so they numb the taste buds and the consumer can't really taste them.

## NUTRITIONAL PROFILE OF SUGAR

Refined cane sugar is a *disaccharide* (double sugar molecule) called sucrose, made up of two single sugar molecules: fructose and glucose. Glucose is the form of sugar the body uses for energy, and in that context it is known as blood sugar or blood glucose. Its levels must remain more or less steady for proper physical function, especially function of the brain, which utilizes about 25 percent of the body's blood glucose.

In terms of actual nutrients, in most refined sugars there is only one: the above-mentioned sucrose. It makes up 99.9 percent of the product. It is entirely lacking in vitamins, minerals, trace elements, fiber, water, protein, fat, and everything else. Nutrients such as chromium, manganese, zinc, magnesium, and copper, all present in the original plant, are lost in the refining process. For that reason, it has been said that sugar provides empty calories. They could be called "naked calories," as well. Brown sugar can be a less refined version of cane sugar if it retains its original molasses and minerals. However, in the United States it's mostly white sugar with some molasses added back into it, much like graham flour is white flour with some wheat germ added back in. The difference between white sugar and brown sugar is the same difference you'd find between a naked man and a man wearing only a tie!

Simple carbohydrates such as cane sugar are quickly absorbed into the bloodstream, where they provide a quick high—and a subsequent crash, or hypoglycemia, when the insulin gets rid of too much blood sugar, giving rise to dizziness and a feeling of weakness. On the other hand, complex carbohydrates such as whole grains or vegetables, because of the presence of fiber and other nutrients, are absorbed more slowly and therefore tend to provide a more even supply of energy, without the big highs and lows.

Currently, sugar has lost some cachet, but instead of slowly disappearing from the marketplace, it is now more ubiquitous than ever. Even products in natural food stores that used to be sweetened with fruit juice, and so were acceptable to me, now are all sweetened with ingredients such as organic cane crystals, evaporated cane juice, turbinado sugar, Demarara, Sucanat, or Florida Crystals. These area all essentially the same thing—highly refined products of the sugarcane.

## SUGAR AND HEALTH PROBLEMS

To focus the issue into a short list, here are some of the health problems associated with sugar, according to nutritionist Robert Crayhon (1994):

- Elevated insulin levels and increased risk of diabetes

- High blood pressure, cholesterol levels, and triglyceride levels, which contribute to cardiovascular disease

- Gallstones

- Obesity

- Mood swings and depression

- Increased stomach acidity

- Migraines

- Weakened immune system

- Depletion of B vitamins, calcium, and copper

- Interference with the absorption of calcium and magnesium, thereby contributing to osteoporosis

In addition, sugar imbalances mineral relationships in the body, causes relative deficiencies of vitamin E, chromium, and copper, and interferes with the absorption of protein, calcium, and magnesium (Appleton 2005). This situation will, of course, interfere with the proper metabolism of bone. Most tellingly for the purposes of this book, a 1998 study at the School of Dentistry at the University of Oulu in Finland found that sucrose is definitely implicated in bone loss and osteoporosis. In this study with rats, two groups of rats were fed identical diets, except one group had sucrose as the carbohydrate, and the other group was given starch. It was found that the breaking strength of bones was considerably lower in the group fed sucrose for both males and the females. In females fed sucrose, the width and weight of the tibias were significantly lower than those of the group fed starches, and concentrations of calcium and phosphorus in the tibias were lower as well (Tjäderhane and Larmas 1998).

There is little doubt that the consumption of sugar is related to dental cavities and even gum disease. Because both of these conditions often appear in those who have osteoporosis and therefore can be a marker for bone weakness, sugar should be kept in mind as a food that can damage the bones as well. One of the major reasons why sugar can damage the bones is because it is acid-forming. Although I mentioned that earlier, it bears repeating. Because of its sweet flavor, most people don't think of sugar as creating an acid condition in the body, but it does. And, as mentioned above, in a diet high in white flour and meat and low in alkalizing vegetables, sugar can be a major bone weakener.

## IS SUGAR ADDICTIVE?

For a long time, when faced with the question of whether sugar is addictive or not, consumers said yes and scientists said no. In every class that I have taught for the past thirty years, whenever I asked my students, "Who feels that sugar is addictive to you?" about 80 percent of the class raised their hands. Scientific papers, on the other hand, generally reject the idea. And yet the concept of sugar addiction remains firmly entrenched in the popular mind.

According to the Society for Neuroscience (2003), data compiled over the past few years now provides support for the idea. It appears that the overconsumption of sweets can share some characteristics with substance addictions. For example, studies of opioids, which are brain chemicals associated with a pleasure response, found that when opioid receptors were blocked, humans with eating disorders like bulimia cut their consumption of sweets in half. And in studies where rats were fed sugar water, the rats exhibited signs similar to drug withdrawal when deprived of sugar. Rats weaned off of sugar kept trying to find more, just like drug addicts keep looking for their fix. Not only that, the rats actually preferred sugar to cocaine!

Perhaps, like many people, you've observed something similar in yourself. Have you ever noticed that if you eat no sugar at all, you don't want any, but if you do eat some one day, the next day you look for a sugar fix again? In my experience, cane sugar certainly is extremely addictive. I don't find maple syrup, fruits, or honey so addictive, but other people with sensitivities and candidiasis may react addictively to any kind of refined sweetener.

By some perverse twist of superb marketing, we have come to believe that sugar-sweetened desserts are essential to having fun, adding a psychological dimension to the addiction. We feed our children this devitalized food because they are socialized to expect it, and we to provide it. As adults, most people like to end their meals with a sugar-sweetened dessert. But despite what we know about the downside of this substance—one that British physician John Yudkin (1972) calls "sweet and dangerous" or, in case we don't get the point, "pure, white, and deadly"—many people still feel that they might be "deprived" if they avoid sugar-sweetened foods. I maintain that, for our long-term health and the strength of our bones, this "deprivation" would be a good thing, just like deprivation of tobacco is now recognized to be good, too.

If you're willing to cut your consumption of sugar, here's a list of foods to avoid because of their high sugar content and other unhealthful ingredients:

- Commercial or homemade desserts, cakes, cookies, candies, and snacks made with cane sugar, high-fructose corn syrup, or artificial sweeteners

- Soft drinks, soda pop, lemonade, and the like sweetened with sugar, high-fructose corn syrup, or artificial sweeteners

- Commercially made salad dressings and condiments that are high in sugars, especially cane syrup and high-fructose corn syrup

- Cold breakfast cereals where sugar is one of the main ingredients

## OTHER SWEETENERS

Most people who like sweets get very unhappy if the ill-effects of sugar are made clear. They want to know what they could use as a replacement. Therefore, I would like to offer some commentary on other sweeteners.

Corn syrup and high-fructose corn syrup (HFCS) are highly processed derivatives of corn. Consumption of HFCS increased 1,000 percent between 1970 and 1990, much more than any other food or food group. Consumption of fructose has been associated with increased obesity (Wylie-Rosett, Segal-Isaacson, and Segal-Isaacson 2004), increases in kidney size (in animal studies; Song et al. 2004), hypertension, metabolic syndrome, insulin resistance, abnormal glucose tolerance, and the development of fatty liver (Fields 1998). Clearly, HFCS isn't a very good product, and it certainly won't help bone strength.

Stevia, made from the South American plant *Stevia rebaudiana Bertoni*, is used as a sweetener by many people who react badly to sugar. Stevioside, a high-intensity sweetener 250 to 300 times sweeter than sucrose, is isolated and purified from leaves of this plant. It has an aftertaste that is noticeable. There has been some concern about the negative effects of large intakes of stevia on the reproductive system of males and on the immune system, as well as whether it may interfere with the absorption of carbohydrates. However, it has been used for a long time in Brazil and in general appears to be safe (Geuns 2003). Here's a thought: If stevia is consumed in its whole, natural state, it is a green leaf. Maybe that's fairly safe. But most of the stevia purchased in natural food stores in the United States comes as a white powder, which means it's highly processed. I feel that if it is so concentrated and refined, it cannot be fully trusted. Unfortunately, the studies and commentary I have seen don't clarify which form has been studied.

Honey is a natural sweetener, especially in its unrefined raw form. Still, it is highly concentrated. I believe it is best used medicinally, a small spoonful in a cup of herbal tea for example, rather than as a regular daily sweetener.

Artificial sweeteners such as saccharin or aspartame, on the other hand, are clearly problematic. First of all, because they offer no calories, they supposedly prevent weight gain by offering taste without substance. In other words, they try to fool the body. But that's not as easy to do as it may sound, and it appears that it hasn't worked. Randolph Nesse, MD, and George Williams, Ph.D., give us a clean rationale in their book *Why We Get Sick: The New Science of Darwinian Medicine*. "Sweetness in the mouth, throughout human evolution, has reliably predicted sugar in the stomach and shortly thereafter, in the bloodstream. It is not surprising that the sweet taste quickly resets metabolic processes so as to curtail the conversion of fat and carbohydrate reserves into blood sugar... If the sugar signal is a lie, there could soon be deficient blood sugar and increased hunger" (Nesse and Williams 1994, 150). The hunger would come from the increase in insulin that the pancreas sends in response to that sweet taste. Because the insulin has no actual new blood sugar to work with, it depletes whatever glucose is available, creating, in a sense, hypoglycemia. And how do people react to this drop in blood sugar? They reach for something sweet to eat!

Sucralose, a new noncaloric sweetener, has become extremely popular. However, it is not without problems. In fact, according to an Associated Press report, "While packages of the artificial sweetener Splenda claim, 'made from sugar, so it tastes like sugar,' one competitor argues that this statement is nothing short of false advertising. In fact, this rival, the Equal manufacturer Merisant Co., has filed a lawsuit against Splenda stating the advertisement should read something a little more like, 'made from dextrose, maltodextrin and 4-chloro-4-deoxy-alpha, D-Galactopyranosyl-1, 6-dichloro-1, 6-dideoxy-beta, D-fructofuranoside'" (Caruso 2004).

To keep things simple, remember that fake foodstuffs are not food, and that the body doesn't like being fooled.

## WHAT DO CRAVINGS FOR SWEETS MEAN?

From my thirty years of experience working with food and diets, I have observed that there are three major reasons why people crave sweets:

1. They're addicted.

2. They don't get enough macronutrients. For example, they don't eat sufficient protein or fats; or, curiously enough, they eat lots of protein but not enough good-quality carbohydrates. Or they don't eat enough food! In short, they're hungry.

3. They have something emotional going on; this seems especially true of cravings for chocolate.

Here are some recommendations for dealing with each of these issues:

1. For addictions, resisting the craving and substituting with bananas, dates, and desserts sweetened with barley or rice malt syrup is what works best.

2. For insufficient intake of macronutrients, making sure to eat enough food, including enough protein and fat, is crucial. Not consuming enough calories, in the misguided notion that low-calorie eating is healthy, creates hunger. Resisting that hunger would only make things worse and increase cravings. This could lead to real malnutrition. It's better to eat good-quality foods and enough of them, rather than not enough and then pig out on the junk food and sweets.

3. For emotional issues, increased awareness and consciousness, perhaps with professional help, are in order, as is the need to acknowledge what the issues are and make peace with them. Chocolate is only a smoke screen.

Of course, the very best way to satisfy a craving for something sweet is with whole foods, where the sugars are packaged together with beneficial nutrients, as nature intended. Here are some healthful choices that will please your sweet tooth:

■ Sweet fruits, such as bananas, dates, figs, and mangoes. These are high in potassium and other trace minerals.

- Sweet vegetables, especially sweet potatoes, yams, pumpkin, squash, and other orange vegetables. These are especially rich in beta-carotene and other antioxidants. Try baked yams as a snack.

- Cookies, cakes, jams, and sweets made with small amounts of natural sweeteners such as maple syrup, agave nectar, or concentrated fruit juices, and, of course, whole grain flours.

- Mineral water or seltzer flavored with apple or other juice.

Bear in mind that a craving for sweets could indicate a deficiency of important nutrients in your diet. Make sure you're getting enough good-quality carbohydrates from whole grains and beans; good-quality fats from extra-virgin olive oil, unrefined sesame and coconut oils, and organic unsalted butter; and, of course, enough protein from beans, nuts, wild fish, or organic eggs, poultry, or meat.

# Caffeine

It is well established that caffeine has a modestly damaging effect on bone mineral density and fracture risk (Hallström et al. 2006). The consumption of caffeine is extremely common in our society. Most people rely on at least one cup of coffee in the morning to wake up. But caffeine is also found in hundreds of other common foods and drinks, such as chocolate chip cookies, soft drinks, and even diet soft drinks, many of which one may not think of as containing caffeine.

Caffeine is found primarily in four natural substances:

- Coffee (even decaf)

- Tea (black, green, and white, but not herbal and not rooibos)

- Chocolate (except white chocolate)

- Mate (a South American herbal tea, pronounced *MAH-tay*)

Foods that contain caffeine either contain one of these four substances as an ingredient or, as in soft drinks and medications, have had pure caffeine added. Here's a partial list of foods and other substances that contain caffeine:

- Regular coffee
- Decaf coffee
- Instant coffee
- Black tea
- Green tea
- White tea
- Instant tea

- Dark chocolate
- Milk chocolate
- Cola drinks
- Diet cola drinks
- Other soft drinks
- Some over-the-counter drugs and headache remedies

- Chocolate syrup
- Chocolate candy bars
- Chocolate cake or cookies
- Chocolate chip cookies
- Chocolate or coffee ice cream

A number of studies have shown that caffeine intake is related to both calcium depletion and fractures. A six-year study at the Department of Medicine of Brigham and Women's Hospital in Boston, which followed 84,484 women aged thirty-four to fifty-nine, found that those who drank five or more cups of coffee daily had nearly three times the risk of hip fractures (Hernández-Avila et al. 1991).

Caffeine consumption increases the excretion of calcium and magnesium through the urine, which indicates bone loss. Young women seem to be able to compensate for this loss by means of increased and more efficient calcium absorption from the intestines. Older women, on the other hand, due to age and hormone-related mineral imbalances, apparently don't compensate as efficiently.

You may wonder what level of caffeine intake is safe. According to a study done at the Department of Family and Preventive Medicine at the University of California at San Diego, a lifetime equivalent of two cups of coffee per day is associated with decreased bone density at both the hip and the spine in older women if they don't also drink milk. (Moderate daily milk consumption, about one glass of milk per day, seems to counterbalance the calcium-wasting effect of caffeine somewhat.) Caffeine consumption is also associated with lower bone mineral density in the femur, but only in older women (Cooper et al. 1992).

The studies that I found all dealt with caffeinated coffee. Because I didn't find any on decaffeinated coffee, I have no data on its effect on the bones. However, my suspicion is that decaf is not much better, as coffee is brewed from beans, which are acid-forming; besides, there still are traces of caffeine in decaf. A study run by *Self* Magazine in March 1996 found anywhere between 2 and 33 mg of caffeine per 8-ounce cup of decaffeinated coffee, depending on the brand or the coffee shop (Williams 1996). For comparison, a cup of regular coffee has between 145 and 272 mg of caffeine.

Until more studies are forthcoming, I would err on the side of caution and consider all forms of coffee, black and green tea, chocolate, and cola drinks to contain caffeine to a greater or lesser degree. And with caffeine, less is better. Caffeine stimulates the fight-or-flight mechanism, in which the body releases adrenaline. For this reason, it does make us alert, but it also accelerates the heart rate and constricts the blood vessels, raising blood pressure.

When people stop using any amount of caffeine, even as little as one cup of coffee daily, most get withdrawal symptoms such as headaches and fatigue, which usually disappear in two to seven days. This withdrawal reaction indicates that caffeine is an addictive drug (Silverman et al. 1992; Greden et al. 1980). Therefore, if you want to stop using caffeine, it's best to taper off gradually. If headache is still a problem, beware of over-the-counter headache remedies. Many of them contain caffeine, so they will stop a headache due to caffeine withdrawal, but they will also prolong the addiction and may, in turn, cause a similar headache when you stop taking the medication.

# Alcohol

Excessive consumption of all forms of alcohol (wine, beer, and hard liquor) is a risk factor for osteoporotic fractures for several reasons. Alcohol abuse is frequently associated with magnesium deficiency; this in turn can cause a lower production of parathyroid hormone and thereby interfere with mineral absorption (Abbott, Nadler, and Rude 1994). In some cases, people who drink too much may ignore food and lose weight; this weight loss also presents an increased risk for hip fractures. In addition, the loss of coordination and incorrect distance judgment that come with excessive drinking can cause falls, which may result in fractures, particularly if the bones are already thin. And finally, a number of studies show that alcoholism decreases bone formation, especially in men (Kim et al. 2003). The good news is that this problem can be reversed within two weeks after complete abstention (Laitinen et al. 1992).

However, with life's perpetual pendulum swing, the situation may be different for postmenopausal women. Researchers with the Framingham Heart Study, a forty-year-long ongoing study of heart disease and its risks in the residents of Framingham, Massachusetts, concluded in their 1988-89 evaluation that alcohol intake of at least 7 ounces per week appears to be associated with higher bone density in postmenopausal women, possibly because alcohol augments the body's estrogen levels (Felson et al. 1995). (For clarity, that means one drink daily, where a drink is 1 ounce of hard liquor, 4 ounces of wine, or 8 ounces of beer.) On the other hand, alcohol might also increase hot flashes! So choose your risk factors wisely.

Alcohol abuse is frequently associated with magnesium deficiency; this in turn can cause a lower production of parathyroid hormone and so interfere with mineral absorption (Abbott, Nadler, and Rude 1994). Magnesium deficiency also is associated with a lower deposition of calcium in the bones.

On the whole, most studies point out the dangers of excessive alcohol intake. Moderation means no more than one drink per day for women and two per day for men. Common sense says that it pays to be safe by using alcohol within these limits.

# Nightshade Vegetables

The concept that the nightshade vegetables affect calcium balance has been put forth for over twenty years by Dr. Norman Childers, a professor of botany at the University of Florida at Gainesville and formerly professor of horticulture at Rutgers University. The nightshades are a botanical classification of plants (Latin family name Solanaceae) that includes many poisonous or medicinal plants, such as deadly night-shade, belladonna, and mandrake. Other members of this family are undoubtedly quite familiar to you: potatoes, tomatoes, eggplant, bell peppers, chile peppers, and tobacco.

According to Professor Childers (1999), nightshade consumption correlates with osteoarthritis because these plants contain glycoalkaloids, which disturb calcium metabolism and tend to remove calcium from the bones, causing aches, pains, and even deformation. Dr. Childers has found that when people with osteoarthritis, joint pain, bursitis, and bone spurs stop using these foods, in many cases their pain and symptoms abate dramatically after four to six months.

Glycoalkaloids are generally poisonous. For example, we find them as nicotine in tobacco, solanine in potato and eggplant, and tomatine in tomatoes. They may also have stimulant properties, as capsaicin (in chile peppers) does. A number of drugs are made from nightshade plants, including scopolamine, atropine, hyoscyamine (Symax), and belladonna (Childers 2002).

My theory is that people eat so many nightshades to counterbalance their consumption of milk products, which have more calcium than human beings need. Consider this: 100 grams of mother's milk contains 33 mg of calcium, whereas the same amount of cow's milk contains almost four times as much: 118 mg. If we assume that the milk of each species is perfectly tailored to the needs of its young, it makes sense that cow's milk has so much more. After all, it's designed to help a calf grow its bones up to cow size—quite a bit more than what a human needs! The calcium in cow's milk, then, is excessive for humans. How do we handle this excess? What I've noticed is that in a dietary system high in dairy, people commonly also eat plenty of nightshades, in classic combinations such as pizza, eggplant parmigiana, potatoes and sour cream, curries and yogurt, and so on. I believe that the nightshades might help in breaking up or neutralizing the excess calcium.

Theoretically, then, dairy and nightshades are opposite and complementary: If you eat one, you need the other. Conversely, if you stop eating one (say, dairy) you might do well to abandon the other, or there may be repercussions on your body's calcium balance. And in fact, many of my students and acquaintances have found that if they keep eating nightshades after adopting a low-fat, dairy-free diet, their joints begin to ache. However, I have noticed that some people are very good at balancing milk products and nightshades. They don't seem to react to either, remaining free of arthritis, joint pains, bone spurs, and other problems related to consumption of both nightshades and calcium. Others are highly sensitive to these plants and feel pains in their joints as soon as they eat even a little. It may even be that the "growing pains" experienced by children and teenagers is associated with their extensive consumption of tomatoes, potatoes, and foods made with them.

Fortunately, aches and pains due to nightshade consumption will reverse in a minimum of ten days and a maximum of four to six months if these foods are removed from the diet. If you really love them and want to eat them anyway, I suggest looking at what the Greeks and Italians have traditionally done for generations: Use the night-shades with plenty of olive oil to balance the taste and small amounts of feta or Parmesan cheese for the calcium balance. While I have no actual data on the effective-ness of this suggestion other than traditional usage, it seems to work very well for the taste buds!

The link between osteoporosis and nightshades hasn't been studied much other than by Dr. Childers. However, a 2005 study from the Department of Family and Community Medicine at the Wake Forest University School of Medicine suggests that the use of smokeless tobacco (also a nightshade, as mentioned above) may be a risk factor for osteoporosis (Akhter, Lund, and Gairola 2005; Quandt et al. 2005). It makes sense, as cigarette smoking is a well-known risk factor, as well (see below).

In any case, it may be sensible to pay attention to the food nightshades because of their ability to affect calcium balance. For those at risk for osteoporosis, an occasional potato or tomato may not cause any trouble; however, it could be a good idea to refrain from relying heavily on these vegetables in the diet. Rather than using potatoes as a major carbohydrate, it would be better to use whole grains such as barley, kasha, brown rice, and quinoa. And instead of using tomatoes or hot peppers to flavor everything, a better choice would be spicy seasonings such as white or black pepper (which aren't nightshades), ginger, and garlic, as well as aromatic herbs such as oregano, tarragon, and marjoram.

## Smoking and Bone Health

In addition to all its other negative effects, smoking has been found to be a risk factor for osteoporosis and fractures, although the mechanism is not yet clearly under-stood (Wong, Christie, and Wark 2007). A review of eighty-six studies found that, compared with nonsmokers, smokers had much lower bone density. The effect appeared to be more noticeable in men than in women, and the elderly were also significantly affected. The study estimated that the lifetime risk of sustaining a hip fracture may be 31 percent higher in women smokers, and as much as 40 percent higher in male smokers. The good news is that quitting can reverse these statistics quite noticeably (Ward and Klesges 2001).

## Citrus Juices and Vinegar

In the section on acid-alkaline balance, I mentioned that fruits are alkalizing because of their potassium content, which is also the case with fruit juices. However, the latter nevertheless may contribute to mineral loss. Citrus fruits are rich in nutrients, as all natural fruits are. Juices, on the other hand, are missing the solids, and with that, important nutrients that balance those in the juice; therefore, drinking the juice may create a relative imbalance. While I've been saying this for years, as an intuitively obvious point, I reiterated it in an interview with *Self* Magazine in July 1995. The author of the article, Diane Di Costanzo, didn't take my word for it and had the pulp analyzed. She wrote, "An analysis of 100 grams of orange pulp discarded from a juice extractor proves Colbin's point: the discarded pulp contains 6 percent of the oranges' vitamin C; 72 percent of the calcium; *all* the folic acid; and 76 percent of the fiber. It's the fiber that may help prevent some cancers as well as stave off energy swings. Fruit juices deliver sugars to the blood like a bullet, creating a spike, followed by a crash. Fiber slows the absorption rate of sugar to the blood" (Di Costanzo 1995, 133).

In some situations, this high amount of sugar, plus the natural acids (indicated by the level of sourness in the flavor of the juice), could affect the body's mineral balance. The same is true for vinegar. The conditions in which this effect could happen are, in my observation, long-term low-fat diets, both omnivorous and vegetarian, as well as low-fat dairy-free diets. And don't forget that the discarded pulp also contains 72 percent of the orange's calcium content! Clearly, it's better to eat the whole orange.

## Weight Loss and Low-Fat Diets

One of the major risk factors for osteoporosis is being too thin. For women especially, this is a problem. Our current aesthetic dictates that you can never be too thin (or too rich, but that's another book). Unfortunately, in terms of health that isn't true. You *can* be too thin, as in gaunt, emaciated, and starved, particularly if you're over fifty. In terms of bone health, being noticeably thin or bony puts both men and women at risk for fractures, particularly when older. According to the National Institute on Aging, women who lose 10 percent or more of their body weight after the age of fifty have twice the risk of breaking a hip as women who don't lose weight (Langlois et al. 1996). As men also get osteoporosis (mostly in association with aging, alcoholism, or malnourishment), the same applies to them: Weight loss after fifty years of age is associated with a higher rates of fracture (Langlois et al. 1998).

Women need between 22 and 27 percent body fat for proper hormone balance. Top models and anorexics may have as little as 10 to 12 percent, and although many of us aspire to the "ideal" they embody, that isn't enough fat for hormone production, or for optimum health. A health professional can measure your percentage of body fat using calipers to measure skin folds. There are also a variety of body fat measurement techniques described on the Internet. People can be too thin from different causes. In our culture, excessive thinness is mostly the result of some type of food restriction, either because of careless, nonnutritious eating, or purposely for weight control, health, or spiritual or political reasons. Strict calorie restriction, anorexia, unbalanced or inappropriate vegetarian diets, and diets high in junk food and refined carbohydrates—any of these can bring it on. (Some diseases that cause malabsorption, such as cancer and AIDS, can also cause excessive thinness or wasting; however, these problems are beyond the scope of this book.)

Much to their chagrin, most women put on weight after menopause even if their eating habits remain the same. Their metabolism can change to such an extent that even fasting or dieting actually increases their weight! Rather than fighting nature, let's look at what's going on; nature has its reasons—and reason can't always second-guess it.

Once the ovaries stop producing estrogen, a woman's body keeps on making small amounts of this hormone in subcutaneous fat, especially abdominal fat. Therefore, the extra weight is actually a good thing for menopausal women, believe it or not. Putting on this weight helps protect the bones not just because it facilitates continued natural estrogen production, but also because the strain of carrying the extra weight is a form of exercise and makes the bones work harder against gravity, thereby helping preserve bone density.

In the extreme, obesity is known to be protective against osteoporosis. But as is usually the case with extremes, it's problematic: Obesity is a risk factor for heart disease and diabetes and calls for a change to a healthier diet. At the very least, people with excess weight would do well to increase the amount of fresh vegetables and fruits in their diet to reach five to seven servings daily.

That a little extra weight might be a healthy thing is an extremely difficult notion for women to accept, as we hear over and over again that we should keep our girlish figures. Impossible! And not even desirable. I think that older women who are excessively thin never look as good as thin young girls. And a little plumpness may just fill in the wrinkles and help us look better. My school friend Elida, after hitting menopause, commented, "At this stage of the game, it's either your face or your butt. I'll take the face anytime!" That said, there are quite a few women nowadays who seem to keep their premenopausal figures, even well into their sixties and seventies. An unscientific survey I have been undertaking seems to indicate that these are all women who have been on hormone replacement therapies since perimenopause, and therefore cannot be said to have truly entered menopause.

Weight loss by fat restriction appears to directly cause bone density loss; therefore, extremely low-fat diets can increase the risk of osteoporosis. In addition, vitamin D, necessary for the absorption of calcium from the intestines, is a fat-soluble vitamin. It is possible, then, that a long-term, chronic deficiency of healthy fats in the diet can contribute to bone thinning because the body can't absorb and retain the necessary calcium due to lack of vitamin D. In his classic book *Nutrition and Physical Degeneration* (1979), dentist and researcher Weston Price mentions the story of a young boy with a leg fracture that hadn't healed in three months. The boy, who had almost constant seizures, subsisted mostly on white bread and skim milk. Dr. Price put him on whole wheat porridge made from freshly ground wheat, whole milk, and a teaspoon of high-vitamin butter with each meal. Within a month the boy's fracture had healed and his convulsions disappeared, and within six weeks he was running and jumping over fences like any normal child. Dr. Price also found that household pets given white bread, sweets, and jams develop malformations of the bones and jaws.

## Lack of Exercise, or an Excess

The bones are designed to move and to function in opposition to gravity. If we deny ourselves that movement—if we mostly sit, ride, take elevators, and avoid walking as much as possible—the bones will diminish for lack of use. Sometimes immobility is unavoidable, as in cases of serious illness or injury where the person is bedridden or unable to move. Bone loss is an inevitable side effect of such conditions.

Children are often prevented from walking and running by constantly being required to sit down and be quiet, in strollers, in car seats, in buses, in schools. These habits of restricted motion may carry over into adulthood and help create the proverbial "couch potato." In her magnificent book *The Continuum Concept* (1986), Jean Liedloff points out that children between birth and about age one are meant to be carried upright, in arms or in a sling, and participate in the movement of their mother's body, rather than being laid down in strollers and cribs. She contends that the absence of that period of being carried, what she calls the "in-arms phase," has lifelong implications. While I am not in favor of children running around in restaurants or at dinnertime, I do believe they need activity. And it could very well be that their hyperactivity at inappropriate times is sometimes an outlet for the many hours of being still or sitting that our social system asks of them.

While activity and exercise are indisputably good for the bones, there is a flip side to this coin. It's that perverse and inevitable pendulum swing, where trouble arises at the extremes. Consider the following facts, which once again illustrate my "three bears rule":

- Lack of exercise or movement causes bone loss.

- Too much exercise or high-intensity athletics causes bone loss.

- Exercise such as walking and weight training promotes healthy bones.

While the first two statements may appear contradictory, all three are true. Female athletes can actually lose their periods because their estrogen production is diminished by the lack of body fat, especially when their body fat is very low, at about 10 to 12 percent. This lack of estrogen in turn causes bone loss. The combination of disordered eating, lack of menses, and osteoporosis has been called the "female athlete triad" (Brunet 2005), although it isn't always female athletes who get it. Male athletes can also experience bone loss due to excessive exercise. For example, a study of a male college division I-A basketball team found that bone mineral content decreased 3.8 percent from preseason to midseason, increased 1.1 percent during the off-season, and decreased another 3.3 percent during the summer months when practice sessions resumed (Klesges et al. 1996).

# Pharmacological Drugs

Our drug culture is pervasive and widespread and permeates every aspect of our lives. I'm not talking about recreational, illegal, or street drugs; those are just the shadow side of the main drugs of our society, the ones sold by prescription or over the counter in numerous legitimate establishments. Several of them directly affect the health of our bones.

## STEROID DRUGS

Steroid and corticosteroid drugs, such as cortisone, prednisone, glucocortisone, glucocorticosteroids, and others of similar names, are used fairly widely in pill, inhalant, or cream form for a wide variety of inflammation and skin irritation complaints, as well as arthritis and asthma. Because they interfere with the absorption of calcium from the small intestine, they can cause bone thinning and osteoporosis, sometimes very quickly. A 1993 study published in the *Annals of Internal Medicine* found that steroids can cause an 8 percent reduction in bone mass (a scale similar to what happens with removal of the ovaries) within four months of use (Laan et al. 1993). In Great Britain, a poll of fifteen thousand users and former users of these drugs found that fully 50 percent had developed osteoporosis. Bone loss from the forearm, for example, can go as high as 10 percent per year in adult subjects taking corticosteroids; as contrast, the normal loss from this site is between 0.5 and 1.5 percent per year after the age of fifty (Pearson and McTaggart 1996).

Steroids are dangerous drugs with well-recognized, serious adverse effects, including weight gain, bruising, cataracts, diabetes, pain in the back and legs, muscle weakness, mood swings, and the well-known "moon face," where the face bloats into a very round form. However, if you're taking steroids and question their role in your bone health, under no circumstance should you just stop taking them. These drugs are often prescribed for serious medical problems, and suddenly discontinuing their use can be very dangerous. Seek the advice of an experienced physician about whether tapering off your use of them is warranted; in addition, your doctor should monitor you during the process of discontinuing the drug.

## ANTACIDS

Over-the-counter, nonprescription antacids are widely used for digestive distress. Their purpose is to *antagonize* the *acids* in the stomach, which supposedly contribute to the discomfort many people feel after eating. A little thought will illuminate what an insane notion that is. The hydrochloric acid secreted in the stomach is essential for the digestion of protein; without it, this process doesn't work properly and protein won't be absorbed. If the stomach is uncomfortable, why target its natural process? Why not change the input so that the natural acids can work properly? Here, as elsewhere, I think of something Dean Black said in his book *Health at the Crossroads*: "Nature has its own laws, and may not allow intrusion without revenge" (1988, 7).

If digestion is uncomfortable, then the practical and sensible things to do to solve the problem would be chewing food thoroughly, changing the diet, and drinking enough water (as opposed to soft drinks). But that's not what most people do, thanks to the relentless advertising of medications for stomach upset, nor is it even what doctors recommend. The treatment of choice usually relies on various over-the-counter or prescribed pharmaceutical drugs.

Antacids work by adding alkalizing substances to the stomach. These drugs are based on either aluminum hydroxide or calcium carbonate. Regarding the former, given the concern with aluminum in the brain of people with Alzheimer's disease, it always comes as a surprise to me that little is said about the aluminum in these and other commonly available over-the-counter drugs. As far as bone health is concerned, aluminum hydroxide antacids (brand names include Maalox and Mylanta) have been associated with bone pain and multiple stress fractures due to phosphorus depletion. Aluminum's dual effect of causing both calcium loss and phosphorus depletion can result in bone loss (Spencer and Kramer 1985). Watch out for aluminum in other medications, too, both prescribed and over-the-counter.

Because of their high calcium content, calcium-based antacids (such as Tums) have become extremely popular as a supplement to ward off osteoporosis. However, calcium supplementation of more than 2,500 mg per day has adverse effects on the balance of minerals in the body (Kato et al. 2004). Recent studies indicate that calcium requirements for both men and women are much lower than had been thought, more on the order of 750 mg per day instead of 1,200 mg per day (Hunt and Johnson 2007). In addition, excessive calcium intake may inhibit the absorption of iron and zinc (Gaby 1994). The condition caused by excess calcium carbonate, called milk-alkali syndrome, is characterized by hypercalcemia (excess calcium in the blood), which can be life-threatening if not caught in time (Addington, Larson, and Scofield 2006). Symptoms include reduction in physical fitness, fatigue, headache, nausea without vomiting, abnormal bone scans, abnormal parathyroid hormone levels, and kidney failure. Medical students have an easy way to memorize the problems associated with this condition: "moans, groans, bones, and stones." Moans and groans because the stones hurt, and bones because they're weakened by abnormal levels of parathyroid hormone (which, as mentioned in chapter 3, is involved in keeping levels of calcium in the blood steady).

With the increased use of these calcium-based antacids as nutritional supplements, hospital admissions for hypercalcemia went from less than 2 percent due to supplemental calcium carbonate before 1990 to over 12 percent from 1990 through 1993, according to a study published in the journal *Medicine* (Beall and Scofield 1995). The condition is reversible if caught early enough and treated appropriately; in some cases, however, permanent kidney damage may occur.

People often take antacids regularly for years without considering possible side effects. I once saw a man for a consultation who had been taking a popular aluminum-based antacid for ten years, twice daily. He had developed amyotrophic lateral sclerosis (ALS, or Lou Gehrig's disease), and I strongly felt that there was a connection between the two. A study published in the *American Journal of Medicine* described a man who had been taking a calcium-based antacid daily for over four years to deal with stomach pain; he had multiple stress fractures, an elevated vitamin D level, and low bone mineralization. In addition, a CAT scan revealed calcifications of his kidneys, which improved somewhat but not totally after treatment (Carmichael et al. 1984).

Taking antacids for alternative purposes, such as preventing osteoporosis, is questionable at best. Considering the actual purpose of these drugs—to affect digestion—it's clear that they will have effects beyond providing supplemental calcium. They will still interfere with the digestion process even in the absence of indigestion. As a result, I imagine that this practice could lead to some type of malabsorption, nutrient deficiency, or the like. And how will this show up? Likely in the form of digestive discomfort and a general feeling that things aren't right. If that isn't attended to, other manifestations of digestive interference may appear. If you are taking antacids as calcium supplements and you don't feel quite "right," consider that there might be a connection. While these drugs, sold abundantly over the counter, may appear benign, remember that, like any other drug, their adverse effects may be quite damaging.

## MALE HORMONES

Androgen-deprivation therapy is a hormone treatment currently being used for prostate cancer. It quadruples the risk of spine, wrist, and hip fractures, which means that as many as 20 percent of the men who are given this treatment may end up with these crippling adverse effects (López et al. 2005). A study published in the *New England Journal of Medicine* found that 19.4 percent of those on androgen-deprivation therapy suffered a fracture, as compared to 12.6 percent in the group not taking the treatment (Tan 2005). Another study, this one from the Department of Urology at the David Geffen School of Medicine and School of Public Health at the University of California, Los Angeles, showed that men with prostate cancer treated with androgen-deprivation therapy were at risk for adverse bone effects from both the disease and the treatment. Fractures were common among this group, with fracture rates higher among those who underwent androgen-deprivation therapy for a longer period of time (Krupski et al. 2004).

## FLUORIDE

For about thirty years, sodium fluoride was used as a treatment for osteoporosis precisely because of its ability to increase bone mass. However, due to findings that it didn't change the fracture rate, this treatment is generally no longer used. Of course, fluoride has other uses, too. Since about 1945, it's been added to municipal water supplies, ostensibly to keep children under the age of six from getting cavities. Essentially, it is a medication that is added to the water supply, with little attention given to the possible problems associated with its enforced consumption. It seems obvious to me that medicating the water supply is not a democratic idea.

There are many health problems associated with fluoridation, such as an increase in uterine cancer mortality, rates of dental fluorosis (fluoride-induced toxicity and tooth mottling) as high as 72 percent in children, lower fertility rates, and osteogenic sarcoma, a type of bone cancer that most commonly affects children. A significant number of studies have found that fluoridated water may in fact increase the rate of fractures, even though fluoride can increase bone mass. For example, one study found that the highest fluoride content in bone ash was found in skeletons of women with the most severe osteoporosis (Alhava et al. 1980).

Fluoride is one of the most toxic elements on earth, and its regular use may impact health in two major ways. The first way is by disrupting enzymes involved in collagen production; collagen is important as the structural protein not just for bones and teeth, but also for ligaments, tendons, and muscles. As discussed, a lack of collagen will lead to brittle bones. The second way fluoride affects health is by damaging enzymes that assist in the repair of DNA, which has effects throughout the body. In addition, fluoride can severely damage the brain, both directly and indirectly. Other toxic effects include dental fluorosis and skeletal fluorosis (when fluoride accumulates in bones, making them extremely weak and brittle). Interestingly, many European countries banned fluoride from their water supply many years ago because research so convincingly linked fluoride to the disruption of collagen formation (Mercola 2005).

Regarding the evidence for the benefits of fluoride, you'd think there would be plenty, given its widespread use. However, this is not the case. Donald J. Miller, MD, in an article titled "Fluoride Follies" (2005), points out that fluoride has long been used commercially as a rat and bug poison, fungicide, and wood preservative. He also states that dental fluorosis is an indicator of fluoride toxicity in the rest of the body and is associated with a lower IQ in children.

A systematic review of water fluoridation studies published in the *British Medical Journal* in 2000 did not find the practice to be safe. As Professor Trevor Sheldon, founding director of the advisory group that conducted the review, explains, "The quality of the research was too poor to establish with confidence whether or not there are potentially important adverse effects in addition to the high levels of fluorosis... The review team was surprised that in spite of the large number of studies carried out over several decades there is a dearth of reliable evidence with which to inform policy"

(Sheldon 2001). The case for fluoride does not stand up to careful evidence-based scrutiny.

Among dentists, there is controversy too. Many support the use of fluoride, both in the water supply and as a topical treatment. Others feel that we are exposed to too much fluoride, and that it is dangerous. According to Susan Rubin, a dentist and holistic health counselor from Mount Kisco, New York, the downside of systemic fluoride outweighs any potential benefits. "Studies point to possible connections to brittle bones [and] increased hip fractures in postmenopausal women in fluoridated communities," she wrote me in August 2005. "There are currently questions of a connection to osteosarcoma. If systemic fluoride had to be approved by the FDA today as safe *and* effective, I do not believe it would be passed. It was implemented in water supplies without ever having to face that type of scrutiny."

She went on to say, "I'm most concerned that a chemical like this is put into water supplies that affect entire populations. What about informed consent? What about medicating entire groups of people who would receive no benefit? Is that ethical? Most people drink fluoridated water without any understanding of the potential hazards. They've only heard the line touted by the ADA and possibly their dentist, and they have not learned both sides of the story... Most of my fellow dentists will not even consider the possibility that fluoride is harmful simply because it is not what we were taught in dental school and the ADA supports water fluoridation. Books, minds and parachutes need to be open in order to work properly!"

There's another wrinkle to this story. According to Mitchell A. Fleisher, MD (2006), who is on the clinical faculty at the National Center for Homeopathy in Nellysford, Virginia, we need to know that fluoride, together with bromides (found in soft drinks, flour in baked good, asthma drugs, and pesticides sprayed on fruits and vegetables) can affect the thyroid. Both interfere with thyroid activity, and their widespread use has coincided with increases of cancer of the thyroid and breast in American women. This is especially noteworthy when you consider that more than 10 percent of the American public has some kind of thyroid problem.

For the health of your bones, and the rest of you, it may be a good idea to avoid fluoridated water, and also fluoridated toothpaste, mouthwashes, and medicines.

# WARNING SIGNS

The body is a rational entity—something we can understand once we learn how to translate its communications. It will not go from perfect health to major illness in a day. Generally there is a slow buildup, or breakdown if you wish, with small complaints and minor symptoms that we generally either ignore or suppress with drugs. Here I'll focus on the small warning signals our body sends us when there is trouble with the skeletal system deep within. Recognizing these signals allows us to take appropriate measures to forestall worse trouble.

Basically, the warning system associated with osteoporosis relates to the structure of the body in general, and to the body's mineral and protein stores. Let's take a look at noteworthy symptoms associated with these nutrients, and where deficiencies may show up first.

## A Bad Taste in the Mouth upon Arising

When you eat acid-forming foods, such as flour, sweets, or protein, without enough alkalizing soups, salads, and vegetables, you may have an unpleasant, sticky-sour taste in your mouth when you wake up, as well as a whitish coating on the tongue. It may be accompanied by bad breath. I always consider this an alarm symptom because it indicates a condition of acidosis, which will eventually draw calcium out of the bones in order to neutralize the excess acids in the blood. Please note that it is almost impossible to test for this, as the metabolic buffering process takes place within minutes. You'll notice that if you do nothing about this taste for twenty minutes or so (no eating, drinking, or brushing), it goes away. That's because the condition will be neutralized by the release of minerals from your bones and/or teeth.

Most people try to fix the bad taste with juice or coffee, and of course by brushing their teeth. However, getting rid of the taste is only half the job. If you're familiar with this bad "morning mouth," experiment with changing your diet. I believe the best way is to wake up with *no* taste in the mouth, and that can be done through careful dietary choices, such as eating more alkalizing vegetables and nonstarchy soups (try vegetable, chicken, and miso soups), avoiding baked and fried flour-based foods (including bread and doughnuts), and not eating desserts based on flour and sugar. This dietary approach is especially important for the last meal of the day. Try eating a dinner without starch, such as fish, salad, nonstarchy vegetables, and a fruit dessert to see how that works for you.

## Hair and Nails

Both the hair and the nails are extensions of the skin and composed mostly of protein. They contain no nerves and therefore have no feeling. However, they aren't "dead"; they're very much alive and constantly growing. At the point where their growth originates—the hair bulb and the nail fold and bed—they are nourished by the blood, so they can easily show the condition of the body's nutrient stores. In severe cases of malnutrition, for example, the hair becomes brittle and can be pulled out with no pain. A diet that alternates between adequate and insufficient protein intake can result in a condition known as *flag sign*, where the hair loses and then regains its pigmentation, resulting in alternating bands of pigmented and white hair.

Dry, dull, brittle hair, and weak, thin, peeling nails can be a sign of insufficient protein intake, a condition that can result from a diet with a high proportion of carbohydrates or a low proportion of fats and protein, or a diet generally too low in calories. As bones need protein for their flexibility, a long-term protein or calorie deficiency signaled by hair and nail weakness can eventually lead to brittle bones, regardless of the intake of calcium. As I mentioned earlier, a lack of water may contribute to these problems as well.

## Teeth and Gums

The wisdom of the body dictates that imbalances will show up first in areas with the least survival value, and then affect progressively more critical systems. In addition, Chinese medicine and other systems of diagnosis consider that the outside is always a reflection of the inside, so that trouble inside the body generally shows up in some sort of external manifestation. As the jaws are part of the skeletal system and teeth need minerals as much as bones do, trouble with the teeth and gums can be an indication of impending or current trouble with the bones. One study found that women with osteoporosis have significantly higher gum recession and therefore are at higher risk of losing their teeth than people with normal bones (Mohammad, Brunsvold, and Bauer 1996). Another study, this one in *Age and Ageing*, found that a decrease in bone density in men was consistently associated with increased tooth loss. Postmenopausal women with osteoporosis also have a higher than expected number of dentures, as well as fewer teeth than women without osteoporosis (May et al. 1995).

Before we get to tooth loss and advanced gum disease, we get other signals. Certain foods seem to have an effect on the teeth, and so possibly on the skeleton in the long run. For example, sour foods such as vinegar, citrus, and tomatoes, when eaten in a low-fat, low-protein diet, can damage the enamel or cause toothaches. The toothaches are usually in teeth already weakened by cavities, even when filled. In my own case, when I had orange juice (freshly squeezed!) every day for a month, one of my wisdom teeth (one with a big cavity) started hurting quite acutely. My dentist had no solution other than an offer to yank out the tooth, which I wasn't ready to do. Instead, I tried to get rid of the pain by following a rather politically incorrect diet for a few weeks: no fruit, no salad, no vinegar, no juices, and plenty of butter and olive oil on everything. I even ate a few good portions of Brie! It worked within a week. Once the pain was gone, I cut down on the fats, was able to eat fruit again sporadically, and ate salads as usual, with modest amounts of dressing. I'm not sure how this worked, but it did.

## Joints and Back

Aches and pains are a warning sign from the body that something needs attention. Taking painkillers to get rid of the pain is sometimes necessary, but you shouldn't stop there. Would you cover up the dashboard of your car to hide a light warning that your brake fluid is low? However, often the problem is that we don't have a good model to help us figure out why there is pain, what it is saying, and what to do about it. If a light went on in the dashboard and it had no explanation, you would probably ignore it or cover it up for lack of knowledge. It is important to try to figure out the root problem causing unexplained pain and then attend to it. Let me give you a few pointers that I have found to be very helpful in diminishing or eliminating minor aches and pains.

For pain in the muscles or joints, there are three dietary factors that should be evaluated:

1.  The intake of raw foods, fruits, juices, sodas, and alcohol *in a low-fat diet*

2.  Intake of nightshade vegetables (tomatoes, potatoes, eggplants, bell peppers, and chile peppers)

3.  A high intake of calcium and vitamin D in supplement form

And here are my recommendations for correcting each:

1.  Either eliminate raw foods, fruits, juices, sodas, and alcohol completely or increase your intake of *healthy* fats. Or perhaps do both, depending on how much your joints hurt.

2.  Definitely eliminate all the nightshades for a few months. Yes, it sometimes takes that long to see results, because the body needs to rebuild itself.

3.  Eliminate the supplements entirely and rely more on nutrient-rich foods.

For pain in the back, first go to a good chiropractor or osteopath. If nothing shows up there, a good deep tissue or shiatsu massage can be helpful in loosening tight back muscles. Chronic low back pain, incidentally, has been considered a risk factor or warning signal for osteoporosis (Ojeda 1995). Heed the warning, change your diet, do more walking, stretching, and gentle yoga, and look at whatever other areas of your life give you a pain in the bottom. Just make sure to face the issue and not deny it, so you can avoid making it worse.

## Stress

When we are under constant pressure, always meeting deadlines and fighting the competition, our adrenal glands, which secrete the fight-or-flight hormone adrenaline, go into overdrive and eventually become exhausted and ineffective. Lack of protein and excess carbohydrate further fuel this process. Christiane Northrup (2006) points out that women who have chronically high levels of the stress hormone cortisol in their bodies are at increased risk for osteoporosis. Stress is also closely related to insufficient sleep, so make sure you sleep well and enough, as this allows your body to repair itself and refreshes your mind as well.

## Other Alarm Symptoms

In her book *Menopause Without Medicine* (1995), Linda Ojeda lists some additional symptoms that may signal osteoporosis well before the bones break, including the following:

- Loss of height (which may indicate collapsing vertebrae)

- Nocturnal leg cramps

- Transparent skin

- Rheumatoid arthritis

- Restless behavior (foot jiggling, hair twisting)

- Insomnia

She says that all of these are indications of lack of calcium or magnesium in the body. Should you find yourself with any of these symptoms, review your diet, your activity level, the medications you take, and the amount of coffee and alcohol you consume. These may signal that it's time to develop new health habits, or to check with a health professional or nutritionist.

# A DIET THAT WILL PROMOTE OSTEOPOROSIS AND FRACTURES

Just to make it perfectly clear, here's a concise list of dietary and lifestyle factors that may increase the risk for thinning and breaking bones:

- Eating a low-fat diet

- Eating refined carbohydrates, such as white bread and pasta, daily

- Eating sugared breakfast cereals with low-fat milk

- Not eating much protein, or eating insufficient good-quality protein

- Eating tomatoes and potatoes daily

- Eating lots of cookies and cake

- Regularly drinking coffee or decaf

- Taking lots of medications, either over-the-counter or prescribed

- Hardly ever going out in the sun

- Doing little if any exercise or walking

Do you know anyone who lives this way?

Now that you know what elements can weaken your bones, you have a clearer view of what you might be doing in that area. As usual, knowledge is power; with this information in hand, it's within your power to make changes that can have a big impact on your health and well-being. In the next chapter, we'll take a look at standard recommendations for strengthening and protecting the bones, and examine some of the pitfalls of the conventional approach.

# CHAPTER 5

# Standard Suggestions for Strengthening Bones: Some That Work and Some That Don't

*It is frightening how dependent on drugs we are all becoming, and how easy it is for doctors to prescribe them as the universal panacea for all ills.*

—Charles, Prince of Wales, 1985 address at the anniversary dinner of the British Medical Association

As mentioned in other chapters, there is a great deal of marketing going on in relation to fragile bone syndrome. While some of the associated advice is sound, much of the marketing—the relentless reminders of what could be wrong with you—ends up creating fear.

Both the National Osteoporosis Foundation (2008b) and the Mayo Clinic (2007) recommend that you engage in weight-bearing exercise, avoid smoking and excessive alcohol, and limit caffeine. However, they really don't say much about what to eat.

Mostly they recommend having bone density tests and taking supplements of calcium and vitamin D, medication, and sometimes even hormone replacement therapy.

Do these recommendations work? Are there any drawbacks to them? Well, it seems to vary: Some of them seem to work ... sometimes. In truth, their effectiveness, and their drawbacks, depend on the person and whatever factors may be involved in that person's situation.

In a 1997 column, Jane Brody, the well-known *New York Times* medical reporter, discussed her friend Helen, who "was certain that osteoporosis was one problem she would not have to worry about. She had been taking estrogen since menopause and calcium supplements for years. She quit smoking decades ago and remained unusually physically active throughout her adult life" (Brody 1997). Already in her seventies, Helen regularly walked for exercise, cycled, played tennis, and, in winter, ice-skated. And yet one day on the rink she collapsed with a broken hip and arm, without having tripped or slipped. In other words, her bones broke simply from gravity, rather than from trauma—a classic fragility fracture.

Unfortunately, Brody went on to assume Helen's problem was due to her not taking the recommended drugs to slow down the loss of bone. I would say that what Helen's unfortunate condition shows is that the currently recommended regime doesn't always work, and I believe that adding more drugs to the mix would be unlikely to make things better. In fact, I wonder whether the current regime of hormone replacement and calcium may actually be making the problem worse, perhaps by some mechanism we haven't yet discovered. Obviously, something is missing from the standard approach.

Here are the standard suggestions that I particularly call into question:

- You must get your calcium from milk products or supplements.

- You should add soy to your diet.

- It's important to have bone density tests.

- It's important to take medication to avoid or slow bone loss.

- Women should use hormone replacement therapy to avoid bone loss after menopause.

Since this advice is currently conventional "wisdom," I don't expect you to just take my word that there are problems with the standard approach. In the rest of this chapter, we'll take an in-depth look at the other side of milk products, supplements, soy, bone density tests, and pharmacological drugs that affect bone modeling, including hormone replacement therapy. In the rest of the book, we'll look at what you can do to strengthen your bones naturally.

# MILK PRODUCTS AND BEYOND

It is common knowledge that milk products are a source of calcium, thanks to the continuous marketing of the dairy industry. However, the recommended milk is low-fat or skim milk. This may create other problems. When the naturally occurring butterfat is removed from milk and other dairy products, these foods are proportionately too high in acid-forming protein. The natural butterfat, together with the calcium, buffers the acidity created by metabolism of the protein; it also helps the body absorb the protein better. There is a reason why nature puts all these nutrients together, and we humans may be quite foolish to think our technology can create a healthier product by removing components of whole foods.

One problem with milk products is that, for many people, they create an excess of mucus. In addition, allergies to these foods are extremely common. In children plagued by colds and ear infections, these complaints often diminish or disappear when dairy products are removed from their diet. The consumption of milk products is also associated with numerous health problems in women, including chronic vaginal discharge, acne, menstrual cramps, fibroids, chronic intestinal upset, and benign breast conditions, as pointed out by Dr. Christiane Northrup in her book *Women's Bodies, Women's Wisdom* (1998). Eliminating dairy foods improves all these problems, as well as endometriosis pain, allergies, sinusitis, and recurrent yeast infections. Here's a simple way to remember the basic concept: Milk should go *out of the woman*, not in. When it goes in, it goes the wrong way and the system jams.

Some studies also find a correlation between juvenile diabetes, ischemic heart disease, and milk intake (Elliott et al. 1999; Laugesen and Elliott 2003). Interestingly, the correlation is not with the milk fat, but with the casein, or milk protein. Thus, low-fat milk doesn't seem to be any better in this regard, and could actually be worse.

In a number of cultures, including those of northern Europe, India, Tibet, and the African Masai, milk products are a natural and traditional food. For these people, dairy products are a healthful alternative, provided that they are produced and consumed in traditional ways. For example, the dairy herd usually consists of healthy animals grazing on natural grass and shrubs. The milk is used in its full-fat form and remains unpasteurized and unhomogenized. In addition, it is most frequently used in fermented or cultured forms, such as yogurt, kefir, and certain cheeses.

In traditional societies other than the few mentioned above, dairy foods are not part of the native diet (Price 1979). Therefore, by about age four most people in the world lose the activity of the lactase enzyme, which digests lactose, and become lactose intolerant. A careful genetic study indicated that the ability of adult humans to digest lactose is a genetic mutation, as it is common mostly in populations that have been using dairy products for millennia (Holden and Mace 1997). An average of 70 percent of adults worldwide are lactose intolerant, but this figure varies widely across cultures. For example, it's only 3 to 5 percent in Scandinavia and 20 percent in Austria, but is as high as 70 percent in Italy and southern India, 80 percent among African Americans, and 90 percent in nondairy cultures in Africa (de Vrese et al. 2001). Clearly, lactose intolerance is not a disease, but the normal state of adult mammals, the class to which we belong. The condition manifests as digestive disorders, stomachaches, bloating, gas, and diarrhea after the consumption of milk products.

For all of these reasons, I generally don't consider dairy products a good-quality source of calcium. So where should we get our calcium? As mentioned in chapter 4, leafy greens are an excellent source, and if you doubt this, just remember that this is where the animals with the biggest bones, such as horses and elephants, get theirs.

And if you're thinking, "Well, I (or my kids) just don't like vegetables," consider this: It could be that the reason you don't like vegetables is because you eat dairy products. Why would this be the case? Because milk is just vegetables that have been processed by a cow. Your body knows you've already had them. Why should you have them twice? Both adults and children who don't consume milk products like vegetables just fine, as I've seen not only with my students, but also with my children and especially my grandchildren, at this writing three and six years old, who eat beets, kale, and spinach out of the garden with great gusto.

If you decide to use milk products, the most healthful ones are organic, raw, full-fat whole milk (without added synthetic vitamin D) and unpasteurized cheese and yogurt made from whole milk from organically raised, grass-fed animals. Cultured and fermented whole milk products, which have lost most of their lactose, are the easiest forms to assimilate.

If you are in a situation where there are few or no vegetables available, and no seaweed, parsley, or calcium-rich soups or stocks, then milk products would be necessary as a source of calcium, provided you aren't allergic to them. If you decide to continue using coffee or nightshades, a small amount of good-quality dairy may be appropriate, as it provides calcium to buffer the alkaloids in coffee and nightshade vegetables.

In the face of the relentless propaganda pushing milk as a good source of calcium and therefore valuable for preventing osteoporosis, let's remember that osteoporosis is more common in dairy-consuming regions such as northern Europe, Canada, and the United States. Not only that, according to a paper on the Nurses' Study in the *American Journal of Pubic Health*, when seventy-eight thousand nurses were followed over twelve years, those with a dietary calcium intake higher than 450 mg per day had *double* the risk of hip fracture, and that was on a standard American diet. What is especially interesting to me is that the high calcium intake was obtained by drinking milk; that is, women who drank two or more glasses of milk per day had a 50 percent higher risk of breaking a hip than women who drank less than one glass per week (Feskanich et al. 1997, 992).

People who consume milk products need to be especially attentive to how this affects their health, including any allergies, colds, recurring bronchitis, ear infections, female disorders, skin outbreaks, digestive disorders, excessive mucus, or being overweight. Because I have seen so many people get rid of those conditions when they started avoiding milk products, I believe that on the whole most of us are better off not using them regularly. For that reason, you will find almost no dairy products in the recipes in part 3, except for occasional use of butter or a little Parmesan or Pecorino Romano. If you consume milk products regularly or use them in your cooking, make sure that they are from healthy cows, as mentioned above. Organic butter from cows that graze on green grass is naturally high in vitamins A and D.

On a spiritual level, let's remember that milk is a baby food. I believe that as long as we drink milk, we are not weaned and we cannot attain our full potential as adults. A continued heavy dependence on milk products may keeps us too close to a childlike emotional state. Becoming weaned off milk is a major step toward self-reliance and empowerment.

## SOY AND ITS SURPRISING RISKS

Since the late 1980s there has been a great deal of emphasis on using soy for women's health issues. Interestingly, that's also about the time that soybeans began to be genetically engineered. I always found this a curious coincidence of timing.

Regular (non-GMO) soybeans are known to contain both phytoestrogens and goitrogens. Phytoestrogens (genistein is one of them) are similar to the female hormone estrogen and thus can have both the positive and the adverse effects associated with estrogen. They may diminish hot flashes in postmenopausal women. On the other hand, studies with rats suggest that genistein may adversely affect development of the reproductive system in both male and female embryos, which may manifest into adulthood as reproductive system disorders (Jefferson, Padilla-Banks, and Newbold 2007; Vilela et al. 2007).

Researchers at the University of Goettingen, Germany, looked at the effects and risks of phytoestrogens or isoflavones and reported that "when administered to isoflavone 'inexperienced' women at the time of menopause, the phytoestrogens appear to share the same effects as estrogen used in classical preparations for hormone replacement therapy, i.e. they may stimulate the proliferation of endometrial and mammary gland tissue with at present unknown and unpredictable risk to these organs" (Wuttke, Jarry, and Seidlová-Wuttke 2007, 150). They further commented that phytoestrogens seem to offer mild protection against osteoporosis. The rationale for recommending soy products is that, being estrogenic, they will have a positive effect on bone mineral density. But remember, fragility or brittleness is the larger issue, and greater density doesn't necessarily prevent fractures. In addition, their estrogenic properties may cause problems, especially for women who need to stay away from excess estrogen, such as those at risk for breast cancer.

That soybeans contain goitrogens (substances that weaken the thyroid) has been known for at least thirty years. I mentioned that in my book *Food and Healing*, which was first published in 1986. This is an issue that is mostly overlooked in the great soy marketing push. When clients who come to me for consultation have any thyroid issues, I suggest that they completely avoid soy, with generally good results. In addition, as a legume, soy in its uncooked state contains trypsin inhibitors, also known as proteinase inhibitors. These substances interfere with the activity of the protein-digesting enzymes trypsin and chymotrypsin. In fact, animals fed raw soybean meal have reduced growth and extensive damage to the pancreas. Cooking helps eliminate most of the trypsin inhibitors (Shils et al. 1994). Therefore, tofu and soy milk, which are uncooked, are poor food choices, for both children and adults.

It is important to remember that, as of this writing, about 89 percent of the soy crop in the United States is genetically engineered, most commonly to resist an herbicide (Smith 2007). Studies show that mice fed genetically modified (GM) soy experience unfavorable changes in the liver, pancreas, and testes (Malatesta, Caporaloni, Gavaudan, et al. 2002; Malatesta, Caporaloni, Rossi, et al. 2002; Vecchio et al. 2004). Fortunately, when their diet was changed from GM soybeans to non-GM, their organs returned to normal (Smith 2007). To be safe, if you choose to eat soy products, it's essential that they be organic, non-GM, and preferably in a fermented form, such as tempeh, soy sauce, and natto (a traditional Japanese condiment with a peculiarly strong flavor that isn't particularly loved by Westerners).

While I have met women who feel that their hot flashes diminished due to drinking soy milk, as a whole I would advise against soy as a food for bone health because of all of the other problems mentioned. There are many other foods that better support overall health, including bone health. We'll take a close look at these foods and how to use them in the next chapter.

# BONE DENSITY TESTS—USES AND LIMITATIONS

The most common technology for measuring bone density is dual energy X-ray absorptiometry (DXA or DEXA), which measures mineral density, although there are other techniques as well. DXA measurements are expressed as T-scores, which compare a person's bone mineral density to a reference standard for healthy young women, which is considered the norm. The result is expressed in terms of standard deviation (SD). According to Susan M. Ott (1994), an associate professor at the Division of Metabolism at the University of Washington in Seattle, the World Health Organization has decreed a T-score of 0.8 as normal arbitrarily, rather than studying the median value of healthy subjects and then coming up with the numbers. By doing so, the organization has placed a lot of asymptomatic, healthy people (mostly women) in the "abnormal" range. The World Health Organization also established a T-score of −2.5 SD (below the norm) for osteoporosis, and −1.0 SD for the milder condition known as osteopenia.

Dr. Ott has been warning for some years that there is insufficient data to predict whether the relative risk of fracture changes with a change in bone mass. An abstract of one of her papers in the journal *Calcified Tissue International* includes the following statements:

There is no doubt that the risk of a fracture increases as the bone density decreases. However, even with a low bone mass, the risk of not fracturing a bone over the next year is over 90 percent. Most of the data suggest that patients with severe vertebral fractures have lower bone mass than those with mild fractures, but some women with similarly low bone mass have mild or no fractures. The weight of the evidence suggests that age has an effect on fracture incidence which is independent of bone mass. Trauma is such a major factor that it is surprising to find almost no studies that have controlled for it. The relationship between bone mass and bone failure is strong, but other factors must also be contributing to the bone failure which, like heart failure or renal failure, is a complex, multifactorial disease. (1993b, S7)

In an editorial in the *British Medical Journal*, Dr. Ott points out that there can be numerous problems with these tests due to the imprecision of instruments, errors in interpretation, and other technical errors. In other words, a single test means relatively little. In addition, she says that the incidence of fracture doubles every decade on the same test reading, so fracture risk has a lot more to do with age than with test results (Ott 1994).

There is a surprising lack of consensus as to how to interpret the results of bone mineral density measurements. A 2002 study published in the *Journal of Clinical Densitometry* found that when comparing seven different types of bone densitometry measurements at different body sites, estimates of fracture risk for individual patients varied almost threefold between testing techniques (Blake, Knapp, and Fogelman 2002). That's a big spread. How can we know which is correct?

Lorna Sass, Ph.D., the author of many cookbooks and winner of the James Beard Award in the healthy foods category, is suspicious. "I am beginning to feel there is something not quite trustworthy about these tests," she told me. "*Everyone* who gets tested is told they're not normal for their age. Then they're told to take drugs or hormones." One of my clients came in very worried after a bone density test showed her bones to be osteoporotic. I asked her if she had fallen recently, by any chance. She said she had indeed fallen off her bicycle. But she hadn't broken anything. "Well," I said to her, "that was your *real* bone density test."

As Sheila Haas, Ph.D., dean of Loyola University Chicago's Marcella Niehoff School of Nursing, commented to me in an e-mail, "Current technology for assessing bone health cannot evaluate resilience, which is critical to strong bones. Bones that are dense but brittle will fracture. Bones that are resilient may be strong even though their density isn't ideal by current standards."

So what's the upshot? While bone density tests might have predictive value from a statistical point of view, they may not be useful for the individual. Screening women under sixty-five has not been shown to help prevent fractures. The National Women's Health Network (2008) recommends that the under sixty-five woman avoid bone density tests. If you were to have a bone density test and it came out "abnormal," it would make sense to start with any needed changes in diet and lifestyle long before considering pharmacological approaches.

# PHARMACOLOGICAL PRODUCTS

The medical model we live by relies greatly on synthetic substances that are purported to maintain or enhance our health. These substances are usually presented in pill form but are also available in the form of syrups, drops, and injections. For osteoporosis in particular, numerous medications and supplements are regularly recommended as prevention. I want to point out that, coincidentally or not, those populations who have more access to drugs and pharmacies also appear to have more osteoporosis than those who still rely mostly on traditional and native diets and healing systems—what we now call alternative or complementary medicine. I believe the coincidence is meaningful.

Considering how clear it is that these pharmacological substances are a double-edged sword, as it is known that *all of them* have adverse effects, I am mystified by the enormous appeal of pills and drugs. Perhaps it is because they seem so magical: "Take this pill, and you'll get better without any effort on your part!" But magic has its price. Drugs may produce the desired effect, and they are also likely to have adverse effects. Both are equal. Both count. We cannot have one without the other. Although we are often told that the benefits outweigh the risks, whether they do or don't greatly depends on the situation, the drug, and the person involved.

## The Issue of Supplements

We know that foods are made up of nutrients—vitamins, minerals, protein, fats, and carbohydrates—and that we need an optimal amount of those nutrients in order to be healthy. Nature has set up the system by which these nutrients are delivered in the best and most accessible form: They come packaged together in certain proportions to each other in the form of whole foods. These are fruits, nuts, leaves, roots, tubers, and other vegetables such as broccoli and cauliflower; foods derived from animals, such as meat, fish, fowl, and eggs; and foods resulting from agriculture, such as whole grains and beans. As discussed above, milk products have traditionally been used by only a few populations.

Although whole foods stood our species in good stead for eons, things changed when food processing was discovered and we developed the idea that we could improve on nature. White flour was made by sifting out the bran and the germ. Although it seemed beneficial that the resulting flour was shunned by insects and rodents, this detail should have given us pause. White table sugar is another "food" completely stripped of all of its most beneficial components, whereas the original cane or sugar beet has, as nature ordained, plenty of fiber and minerals.

After a few decades of consuming refined flour and sugar in the nineteenth century, we discovered vitamins, and by the early twentieth century most of them had been found and named. Soon they were being extracted and sold separately. I remember in the 1950s there was so much excitement about concentrating the "active ingredients" out of foods that there was talk of a "lunch pill." We wouldn't have to bother with eating anymore!

Well, the "lunch pill" idea never really took hold, and for good reason. There is so much more to food than the nutrients we can chemically extract from them: protein, carbohydrates, and fats, for one thing—the nutrients that provide us with calories! And, of course, there is the bewildering and ever-expanding array of phytochemicals—nutrients found in plant foods that have powerful health benefits. It's also likely that there are plenty of other nutrients in food that we haven't discovered yet. And beyond the physical, chemical constituents of various foods are their flavors, aromas, textures, and that certain feeling of having enjoyed a good meal—none of that would be available in a "lunch pill."

It is clear that there are cases in which individual nutrients do have a medicinal value, especially for people who routinely consume conventional, refined, processed foods. Vitamin C definitely helps prevent or cure scurvy, a disease common in those who eat no fruits or vegetables. B vitamin supplements are effective against beriberi and pellagra, which develop when people subsist on polished white rice or degermed cornmeal, respectively. Numerous studies as well as multitudes of popular books point out the many benefits of individual nutrients for a vast array of conditions. This information has been extrapolated into the idea that taking various vitamins and supplements is essential to good health, a concept now firmly established in our culture. Unfortunately, this is not always the case.

The ability to digest food and absorb nutrients varies from person to person. Nutrients are absorbed through the wall of the small intestine, which is about twenty feet long. It is lined with small extensions (think of the loops on a terry towel) called villi, which in turn are covered with extensions called microvilli. If you were to flatten everything out, you'd end up with a surface about the size of a tennis court (Lipski 1996). When functioning optimally, this system is very effective. However, some common conditions can lead to malabsorption of nutrients:

- Inadequate chewing

- Eating too many refined and processed foods

- Diseases of the small intestine, including celiac disease, candidiasis, irritable bowel syndrome, leaky gut syndrome

- Antibiotic use, which destroys the intestinal flora

Processed and refined foods can, over time, leave undigested residues along the digestive tract that eventually prevent the absorption of many nutrients. Diseases of the small intestine, such as celiac disease or sprue (the inability to tolerate gluten) frequently result in the malabsorption of vitamin D and minerals. Antibiotics damage the intestinal flora responsible for the synthesis of B vitamins and other nutrients, thereby making these nutrients unavailable for absorption from the bowel (Crayhon 1994). In these cases, careful and *individualized* nutrient supplementation may be in order. In other words, each person's nutritional supplementation regime must be prescribed, after a thorough health history and appropriate tests, by a trained health practitioner. Self-prescription of drugs or supplements is inadvisable. We can cause as much damage by having too much as we can by having too little.

I believe that one of the drawbacks of supplementation is that it bypasses the body's natural efforts to draw nutrients out of food and thereby creates an atrophy of sorts. As the old saying goes, "Use it or lose it." If we get used to natural foods that have the nutrients hidden in the cells, our digestive system becomes quite adept at pulling them out and absorbing them. If, on the other hand, we continuously feed our bodies with readily available nutrients in pill form, one or two things may happen: The body may become lazy and lose the ability to absorb nutrients from food, thereby becoming more and more deficient even in the presence of nutritious foods. Another possibility is that the body doesn't break down the pill so it passes right through, wasting both money and energy.

On a spiritual level, taking supplements without real medical need is based on the emotion of fear, particularly the fear of not having enough. If fear is the motivating factor, perhaps it would be more effective to address that deep-seated feeling than douse ourselves with pills. I prefer to trust that there will be enough of what we need for all of us, although, of course, we need to be conscientious about our choices. Let's remember that in going for the apparent benefit in a straight line, we may once again be generating unintended secondary consequences and causing ourselves unexpected troubles. Taking calcium supplements is a case in point.


## CALCIUM SUPPLEMENTS—ARE THEY REALLY NECESSARY?

Calcium is the main supplement recommended to prevent and slow down osteoporosis. Do we really need it in pill form? Leo Lutwak, MD, in his book *The Strong Bones Diet* (Lutwak and Goulder 1988), points out that many women who take daily calcium supplements may develop abdominal discomfort, constipation, or even kidney stones and not realize there's a relationship. "There are advantages to getting your calcium from foods instead of pills," Dr. Lutwak writes. "Bone health depends not only on calcium, but on many other nutrients that are contained in different kinds of foods" (Lutwak and Goulder 1988, 12). He goes on to point out that foods high in calcium also contain numerous other vitamins and minerals, that vegetables high in calcium are fine sources of fiber, which prevents colon cancer and contribute to satiety as well, and that foods provide energy, while isolated vitamins and other nutrients don't. And, perhaps most sagely, he observes that while you may forget to take your pills, you generally won't forget to eat.

There is much more uncertainty about taking calcium supplements, that seemingly universal recommendation, than one would suspect. Unfortunately, those with a vested interest in marketing milk products and calcium supplements as preventers of osteoporosis continue do their best to keep us purchasing their products. So perhaps our fixation on this conventional wisdom isn't surprising. After all, it also took some time for people to figure out that the world wasn't flat.

## HOW MUCH CALCIUM DO YOU NEED?

In the United States, the official recommendation for intake of calcium is 1,000 to 1,300 mg daily (Institute of Medicine 1997). However, in 1962 the World Health Organization recommended only 400 to 500 mg per day; at that level, people in third-world countries on their native diets did not have the high rate of fractures found in more developed countries (Nordin 2000). In South Africa, rural Bantu women have one-tenth of the hip fractures of Caucasian women, yet they consume only half the calcium (250 to 400 mg daily), even into their ninth decade. On average, the Bantu women studied bore on average six children and breastfed them two years, whereas the white women bore two children and fed them formula diets (Watkins, Pandya, and Mickelson 1985). Why such a discrepancy in fracture rates?

The reason may be found in the women's overall diet. Context counts. In June 1994, the Consensus Development Conference on Optimal Calcium Intake, sponsored by the National Institutes of Health, recommended as much as 1,500 mg of calcium daily for women over fifty who aren't taking estrogen. However, in the same conference, Dr. Robert P. Heaney, of Creighton University in Omaha, pointed out that the amount of sodium and protein in the diet are crucial variables affecting the amount of calcium needed (National Institutes of Health Consensus Conference 1994). When the diet is low in sodium and protein, the daily calcium requirement for an adult female may be no higher than 450 mg, much closer to the amount recommended earlier by the World Health Organization, and an amount easy to obtain from a mostly plant-based diet of beans, grains, and vegetables, with small amounts of animal foods, which is what most traditional people in the world have historically eaten (and the system on which the recipes of this book are based).

If you need further convincing, a paper published in 2000 in the *American Journal of Clinical Nutrition* pointed out that hip fracture rates in many developing countries are much lower than in the West, even though calcium intakes in these countries are typically quite a bit lower (Nordin 2000). For example, in Gambia average daily calcium intake is 360 mg, but osteoporotic fractures are rare. Because the proportions of calcium, sodium, protein, and other nutrients in the diet varies greatly from culture to culture, and from person to person, it must be concluded that there is no single, universal calcium requirement applicable to all individuals (Nordin 2000).

In terms of nutrients, calcium included, it pays to remember my "three bears rule": *Too little* is no good and *too much* is no good; you want to get it *just right*. In other words, if a deficiency is bad, an excess is not necessarily better; in fact, an excess can be bad too. Again, moderation is the key. Yet popular belief that insufficient calcium is unhealthy for the bones often encourages excessive supplementation. According to Nan Kathryn Fuchs, who holds a Ph.D. in nutrition and edits the *Women's Health Letter*, too much calcium can encourage calcium deposits in soft tissue such as the joints, arteries, kidneys, muscles, and brain, and also contribute to kidney stones and gall-stones (Fuchs 2003). Excess calcium may also contribute to an increase in the risk of cardiovascular mortality (Bellinghieri, Santoro, and Savica 2007), and supplementa-tion has been associated with an increased incidence of heart attacks and strokes in postmenopausal women (Nainggolan 2008).

Sue Hitzmann, an exercise physiologist teaching in New York who also regularly performs cadaver dissections, mentioned in a class I took that an older woman she had dissected the week before had calcium deposits throughout her body. "We find calcium deposits in many layers of the body...not just near the bones like you would see in a bunion, but in the connective tissue layers and in between joints," she wrote to me in an e-mail in 2007. Interestingly, a 2005 study in Japan found that calcium and magne-sium deposits in the ligaments of the neck increased progressively with aging (Utsumi et al. 2005). Perhaps this has a bearing on the dowager's hump sometimes seen in older adults. What all these deposits do show, I believe, is that often the excess calcium that people consume, whether from dairy or from supplements, ends up deposited in areas other than where it's wanted—in the bones.

Excess calcium also makes the bones more brittle, a fact that makes sense if you consider that calcium provides hardness and density, but not flexibility. It's flexibility, provided by the collagen matrix or protein, that keeps the bones from breaking. Bones that are hard and dense (high in calcium) but not flexible (because of being propor-tionately lower in collagen) may shatter with a blow. And in fact, a study published in the *American Journal of Epidemiology*, offers support for the idea that calcium supplements often do more harm than good, even for the bones, as they were associated with a dou-bling of the risk of hip fractures, and use of a popular brand of calcium antacids led to a 70 percent increased risk of forearm fractures (Cumming et al. 1997).

Excess calcium—out of its natural context, that is, in supplement form—can cause other problems. The mechanism of muscle contraction, which among other things is important for the continued regular beating of the heart, depends on balanced levels of minerals. When excessive calcium disrupts this equilibrium, it can cause the abnormal heart rhythms and chest pains of heart disease, which is often treated with a class of drugs called calcium channel blockers. According to Ruth Winter (1995), a medical writer and author of many books, calcium supplements and calcium-based medications may cause stomach bleeding, nausea, vomiting, excessive thirst, or abdominal pain, and should be used with extreme caution by people with heart or kidney disease.

As quoted at the start of this book, "Purposeful behavior itself is often counter-productive." When we look at only a small part of the picture (calcium in this case) and lose sight of the whole (the importance of mineral and nutrient balance, and potential problems associated with supplements and consumption of dairy products), we may cause unexpected outcomes. If we remember that a bone high in calcium but low in the collagen matrix is more likely to fracture, it seems to me that the admonition to keep piling up the calcium without attention to the bigger picture could, in fact, be totally counterproductive.

Nature protects us from excess and imbalance by building checks and balances into foods. As we saw in chapter 2, an excess of calcium creates a relative deficiency of magnesium, and may create symptoms associated with those deficiencies. We also need magnesium and vitamin D to absorb calcium properly. The key is to consume calcium *within its natural context*, together with magnesium and all of the other nutrients it naturally co-occurs with. That is how our bodies are programmed to absorb and utilize all nutrients. Whenever we take one nutrient out of context and consume large amounts of it, we become relatively deficient in the all other nutrients that assist in its assimilation.

Alex Vazquez, a naturopathic physician practicing in Seattle and elsewhere and former adjunct professor of orthopedics and rheumatology at Bastyr University, has a very important caveat about use of supplements. In a paper entitled "The Clinical Importance of Vitamin D (Cholecalciferol): A Paradigm Shift with Implications for All Healthcare Providers," he writes that nutritional effectiveness "depends on synergism of diet, lifestyle, exercise, emotional health, and other factors... Single intervention studies are a reasonable research tool only for evaluating cause-and-effect relationships based on the presumption of a simplistic linear model that is generally inconsistent with the complexity and multiplicity of synergistic and interconnected factors that determine health and disease... Optimal clinical results with individual patients are more easily attained with the use of multicomponent treatment plans that address many facets of the patient's health" (Vasquez, Manso, and Cannell 2004, 34).

This is wise counsel. Give it careful consideration before you rush into buying a bag full of supplements.

## Hormone Replacement Therapy and Its Risks

As mentioned in chapter 2, female hormones promote the deposition of bone matter. As estrogen wanes with menopause, women lose the benefits of this particular contributor to bone health. If we do nothing else, and if we consume mostly acid-forming substances such as sugar, coffee, meat, pasta, and bread, our bones will indeed become thinner. But is trying to turn back the clock through use of supplemental hormones really the answer? What are the unintended secondary consequences, or, as they are more commonly known, the side effects of this particular practice?

While hormone replacement therapy (HRT) may result in a temporary slowdown in bone loss, after it is stopped bone loss accelerates, almost as if to catch up with the normal rate, according to an article by Lynne McTaggart in *What Doctors Don't Tell You* (Pearson and McTaggart 1996). She states that among eighty-year-old women, those who took HRT for ten years after menopause are likely to experience about 27 percent bone loss; for women who never took HRT, the figure would be just 30 percent—

hardly a striking difference. Because most hip fractures occur after the age of seventy-five, HRT doesn't appear to be a good preventative measure, unless a woman is willing to take it for the rest of her life—and risk other problems it may bring.

Estimations of the risks associated with HRT vary. It is generally accepted that women on HRT have a higher risk of breast and endometrial cancer (Biglia et al. 2007). The Women's Health Initiative, a large randomized trial investigating the effects of conjugated equine (horse) estrogen plus progestin, found numerous adverse effects of this HRT regimen, including increased breast cancer and dementia (Shumaker et al. 2003). On May 31, 2002, after a mean of 5.2 years of follow-up, the data and safety monitoring board recommended stopping the trial of estrogen plus progestin because the risk for breast cancer, heart disease, and other health problems exceeded the expected benefits (Rossouw et al. 2002). In other words, the results of using conjugated estrogen plus progestin were bad enough that this very expensive trial was stopped. Nevertheless, numerous women remain on HRT, in spite of the data.

Among the documented risks of hormone replacement therapy you can find the following (Runowicz 2003):

- Increased risk of endometrial cancer

- Premenstrual symptoms, including swelling, bloating, breast tenderness, mood swings, and headaches

- Vaginal bleeding

- Increased risk of breast cancer

- Stimulation of the growth of uterine fibroids and endometriosis

- Increased risk of gallstones and blood clots

- Possible weight gain

Be aware that HRT in general is a complex issue, and beyond the scope of this book. There is some suggestion that the synthetic versions of the hormones used in the Women's Health Initiative study may have been problematic. Perhaps bioidentical hormones, which are exactly like the forms that naturally occur in our bodies, would have different results. In any case, our concern here is bone health, and it seems fairly clear that using sex hormones to affect the function of bone is a bit far-fetched. Professor John A. Kanis, of the University of Sheffield Medical School in Great Britain, published a study in the journal *Bone* questioning the logic of giving hormones to women at risk from osteoporosis at the time of the menopause, when most of the risks and benefits of HRT have nothing to do with the skeleton (Kanis 1996). Because of their wide-ranging and possibly adverse effects on other body systems, it may not be wise to take them for the simple purpose of reducing osteoporosis.

In one of those perverse twists that life's pendulum swing often brings, a study published in the *Journal of the American Medical Association* found that women with denser bones have a 2 to 2.5 times *higher* chance of developing breast cancer than women with lower bone mineral density. The authors of the study called for identifying a common denominator for these disheartening statistics (Cauley et al. 1996). However, Lynne McTaggart pointed out that this study neglected to factor in the use of HRT, which is known to increase bone mass and also to increase the risk of breast cancer. Why do the women in this study have higher bone mass? It could be because of exercise, good diet, or, not improbably, the use of hormone replacement therapy (Pearson and McTaggart 1996). Surely the authors of the study should have known that particular variable. As HRT both increases the risk of breast cancer and thickens the bones, we now have a situation not unlike stealing from Peter to pay Paul: Synthetic hormones take away from health in other areas, such as resistance to cancer, in order to benefit the skeleton.

Hormone replacement therapy has been sold to women by tapping into their fear of aging, a fear embedded into our consciousness by the modern culture of youth. It is foolishness—or worse—to try to reverse the process of aging. There is nothing wrong with aging itself. As we get older, there are many mistakes we don't have to make again, many insecurities we can give up, many dangers we can laugh away. And aging does not invariably mean illness and broken bones; there are plenty of older people in their seventies and eighties who are in fine shape and excellent spirits, and who don't routinely fracture. Of the people I know in this age group, those who are healthiest are those who have remained most physically and mentally active. A simple thought experiment will reveal the problem with the idea that broken bones are a result of "estrogen deficiency": *All* women have lower estrogen levels after menopause, but only a minority of them get fractures. I believe that these are more often than not the result of poor lifestyle choices, overall weakness, ill health, or prescription drugs.

We may also want to consider the symbolic and spiritual aspect of HRT. What is the background emotion? Here, too, fear rears its ugly head: the fear of not embodying the cultural ideal, not being attractive, desirable, sexy, or "feminine." It's understandable that we'd have a fear of getting older, heavier, and slower; after all, this type of image is never presented in our media as a desirable or valid stage in a woman's life. Add to that the fact that many older people are sequestered in retirement communities, and therefore the reality and complexity of aging is hidden from us. How much we lose when we aren't connected with that part of life! The images I grew up with, on the other hand, from my mother and other European relatives, friends, and acquaintances, is that older women looked so good, were so together, and knew how to handle life so well that I was actually quite impatient to get to being "older." In fact, I don't think I ever felt I was quite old enough until after I turned fifty.

According to Carol Ellis, MD, a general practitioner in New York City, the long-term use of hormone replacement therapy is still controversial among physicians (personal communication). On occasion, there may be valid medical reasons for its temporary use, perhaps to treat such conditions as severe hot flashes or sleep disturbances. However, considering the attendant risks of cancer and other health problems, using these powerful drugs to prevent bone loss is questionable to say the least, especially considering how many other, less dangerous options we have.

# Drugs to Halt Bone Resorption

Often I get the impression that in our search for health we tend to look for the miracle cure, the magic bullet—or rather, the magic pill. All too often, this impulse leads us to conventional Western medicine and its pharmaceutical solutions because few of us are willing to consider the work involved in changes in lifestyle and other efforts such as "alternative" modalities. In addition to offering the allure of an "easy" treatment, drug medicine is, in fact, extremely effective at finding substances that manipulate and maneuver the body to do one thing or another. Granted, medications may at times be necessary for certain illnesses, and can be very helpful in cases of crisis. However, as many of us have personally experienced, chronic use of drugs often creates a backlash because they tamper with the natural order—something their promoters consistently push as far into the background as they legally can.

The newest miracle cure for osteoporosis is the bisphosphonate class of drugs, such as alendronate (Fosamax), etidronate (Didronel), ibandronate (Boniva), pamidronate (Aredia), risedronate (Actonel), tiludronate (Skelid), and zoledronate (Zometa). (I love the creativity in the names!) These are prescribed to increase bone density and prevent bone loss, which they accomplish by interfering with the process of bone resorption; that is, they stop the bone from releasing calcium and minerals into the bloodstream. In technical terms, they slow down bone turnover. That means it's rather like putting a freeze on withdrawals from your calcium bank. Because the body is still allowed to deposit calcium in the bones, this leads to bigger bank accounts, in the form of bigger bones. And in fact, these drugs seem to increase bone density and decrease the risk of fracture by over 40 percent.

As always, there are adverse side effects to these drugs, which have caused many a user to stop taking them. They appear to cause serious burning in the esophagus, a type of heartburn that doesn't respond to antacids. According to Carol Ellis, MD (personal communication), these effects may be lessened by taking them with a glass of water on an empty stomach, without taking anything else and while remaining upright, maybe walking or riding a bicycle, for thirty minutes. I've spoken to a number of women who couldn't continue taking these drugs because of the side effects. Others had no problem.

So here we have a type of drug that seems to provide a measurable health benefit. However, knowing that to every action there is a reaction, I have two big questions: First, if this drug burns the esophagus to such an extent when it is taken, what else will it burn as it moves through the body? And second (and more worrisome), if you can't withdraw your money from the bank, eventually you'll run into problems with the landlord and the phone company, to say the least. And if you can't withdraw calcium from your bones to maintain the acid-alkaline balance of your blood and handle the needs of your heart, muscles, and nerves, how is that going to affect the rest of your body? Surely this deficiency will eventually make itself known. How long will it take? Will we be able to correlate, say, muscle tremors, if caused by low blood calcium, with the use of these drugs without it being ascribed to coincidence or some other "disease"?

I have asked these questions, rhetorically, in many of my classes on eating for healthy bones. I wondered if taking these drugs would affect heart function especially. I had a hunch that these drugs could affect the heart by preventing the release of calcium from the bones to keep the blood's pH balanced. One of my students recounted the story of his mother, who was in her early seventies and didn't have a preexisting heart condition, yet died of a heart attack shortly after starting on a drug regime to prevent osteoporosis. This anecdotal report proves nothing, of course, yet I found it suggestive. Interestingly, my hunch appears to be correct: In 2007, a paper in the *New England Journal of Medicine* described increased rates of serious atrial fibrillation in patients who took bisphosphonate drugs for osteoporosis (Cummings, Schwartz, and Black 2007). It is also suggestive that in a television commercial recommending this drug, the adverse effects warning for people who shouldn't be taking it included *having low blood calcium*. (If you watch a TV commercial for any drug, close your eyes and listen carefully; they all have to tell you the adverse effects, but you may not notice because of the appealing images, which override the words.)

Professor Susan Ott points out that while these drugs increase bone density in postmenopausal women by about 5 to 10 percent over one year, after that the density appears to plateau because bone formation stops if resorption is halted, so no new bone is made (Ott 1993a). In addition, the long-term effects of interfering with the remodeling cycle are still unknown. The bones themselves might be the victims of subtle side effects, which could go undetected, as bone pain or fractures are usually attributed to the underlying osteoporosis. In fact, in January 2008 a bulletin from the U.S. Food and Drug Administration warned about the possibility of severe and sometimes incapacitating bone, joint, or muscle pain in people taking bisphosphonates:

> Although severe musculoskeletal pain is included in the prescribing information for all bisphosphonates, the association between bisphosphonates and severe musculoskeletal pain may be overlooked by healthcare professionals, delaying diagnosis, prolonging pain and/or impairment, and necessitating the use of analgesics.
>
> The severe musculoskeletal pain may occur within days, months, or years after starting a bisphosphonate. Some patients have reported complete relief of symptoms after discontinuing the bisphosphonate, whereas others have reported slow or incomplete resolution. The risk factors for and incidence of severe musculoskeletal pain associated with bisphosphonates are unknown.

While bone treated with bisphosphonates may become more dense, it also becomes much more brittle. A recent letter to the editor in the *New England Journal of Medicine* of the week of March 20, 2008 described unusual fractures of the hip in postmenopausal women taking alendronate (Fosamax). Two-thirds of the patients were found to share a unique X-ray pattern that isn't commonly seen, particularly in low-trauma fractures. The authors recommended that everyone prescribing these medications become aware of this problem (Lenart, Lorich, and Lane 2008). These kinds of fractures seem to be increasing. Even as this book was going to press, a report in the *New York Times* reviewed several studies of fragility fractures of the upper thighbone in women who have taken these drugs for five years or more. Patients reported that the femur simply snapped after a long period of unexplained bone pain. One source estimated that 5 percent of women taking the drugs might be affected, a not insignificant percentage (Parker-Pope 2008).

Another very serious condition that has emerged as an adverse effect of these drugs is osteonecrosis of the lower jaw, meaning development of necrotic or dead bone in the mouth due to the blood supply to the bone being blocked. Clinical features include local pain, swelling of soft tissue, and/or loose teeth, as well as softened and exposed jaw bones (García Sáenz et al. 2007; Ruggiero and Drew 2007). Dentists call this problem "fossy jaw," a designation that seems to have taken hold (Abu-Id et al. 2008).

Encouraged by their physicians, many women have taken these drugs since they came out in the mid-1990s, unwittingly taking part in something called "postmarketing surveillance," a term that means users of the drug will be monitored, either formally or informally, to see what other good or nasty effects could come from the broader use of it. Knowingly or unknowingly, all of these women are participating in a large drug trial. On top of it, they (or their insurance company) are paying to be part of it. Some results, as mentioned above, have already come in. Not all users will suffer from the side effects of these drugs, but others will, and there's no way to know who will and who won't ahead of time. Is this a gamble you're willing to take?

Now that we've examined the shortcomings of some of the conventional approaches to bone health, let's take a look at what you can do to turn the corner. Believe me, it's not so hard, and it certainly is within your power to make changes that will strengthen your bones from now on.

## PART 2

# Caring for Your Bones

*Bhrigu meditated and found that food*
*Is Brahman. From food are born all creatures,*
*By food they grow, and to food they return.*

—Taittiriya Upanishad, translated by Eknath Easwaran

# CHAPTER 6

# The Whole Foods Approach: How Diet Can Promote Healthy Bones

*When diet is wrong, medicine is of no use.*
*When diet is correct, medicine is of no need.*

—Ancient Ayurvedic proverb

This chapter takes a close look at how to use food to strengthen the bones. As eating is something we all need to do several times a day, it is possible to set up a regular system of choosing healthful, bone-strengthening foods that little by little becomes a full-time habit. I encourage you to create such a dietary program for yourself, even if you start with only 10 percent of what I suggest. A little is better than nothing! Of course, in the long run you need to do more. So as your first round of changes becomes familiar and habitual, revisit your program and make further changes. Ultimately, for optimum bone health you should aim to adhere to these recommendations about 60 to 70 percent of the time. Remember also that if you have a regime that is, say, 70 percent really healthy, occasionally falling off the wagon isn't going to make much of a difference in the long run, although in the short term you might notice some adverse effects. (For details on specific nutrients, see chapter 3.)

# GETTING THE MOST NUTRITIOUS FOOD

In the natural order, we can get all of our necessary nutrients, in balanced proportions, from the foods that nature provides. Before the rise and expansion of Western "civilization," most traditional societies had well-balanced diets based on locally abundant, nutritious foods on which they lived for many generations. For example, at the archaeological site of Ceren, in El Salvador, a village from about 560 AD preserved in volcano ash, there is evidence of abundant food such as corn, several kinds of beans, squash, chile peppers, avocados, nuts, and fruits. Animal proteins were obtained from deer, ducks, dogs, and freshwater mollusks (Wilford 1997). Weston Price, whom I have mentioned before, invariably found that native populations on their original diets had fine teeth, strong bones, and excellent health. But when those same groups came into contact with explorers and missionaries who exposed them to processed and refined foods, such as white flour, white sugar, and canned vegetables, they developed dental problems and within one generation showed malformation of the bones and teeth (Price 1979). Arnold de Vries, in his book *Primitive Man and His Food* (1952), surveyed accounts of voyagers, missionaries, and explorers from the sixteenth century to modern times and found accounts of healthy and vibrant native peoples worldwide, in the Americas, Europe, Asia, Africa, Australia, and New Zealand.

In these modern times, food quality is not nearly as good as it had been for thousands of years. I believe there are three angles to this problem:

1.  **Poor soil:** The land has been overfarmed and depleted by monoculture, and the soil has been damaged by the use of artificial fertilizers, pesticides, and herbicides, often derived from petroleum.

2.  **Poor food quality:** The majority of commercial foods, which are so heavily promoted and widely available, are refined, stripped of their natural nutrients, canned, frozen, artificially colored, artificially flavored, contaminated with thousands of different chemical substances, or otherwise rendered unhealthful.

3.  **Poor health:** Many people are unable to absorb fully the nutrients from the food, mostly because of problems in the digestive tract.

Fortunately, a number of strategies can help us overcome these three factors. Let's take a close look at the solutions for each.

# Combating Poor Soil: Choose Organically Grown or Raised Foods

Organic crops are grown without artificial fertilizers or pesticides in soil that has been free of these chemicals for at least three years and is enriched with organic compost. Organically raised animals aren't treated with antibiotics or growth hormones and are given natural feed or, even better, raised on pasture (grass fed). Organic foods are generally available in farmers' markets and natural food stores, and increasing numbers of supermarkets are carrying them as well. "Organic" is a legal term and comes with strict guidelines. Unfortunately, some elements of the agriculture industry keep trying to weaken the standards.

Beyond being more environmentally sound, organic agriculture and animal husbandry also produce food that's more nutritious. Traditional organic farming methods use compost and manure to return a rich mix of nutrients to the soil, whereas commercial fertilizers add only a few specific nutrients. Tests have confirmed that organically grown vegetables are more nutritious—in some cases as much as 50 to 150 percent higher in nutrients than commercial produce. For example, a review study in the Journal of Agricultural and Food Chemistry found that organically grown tomatoes contain between 79 and 97 percent more flavonoids than those grown commercially (Daniells 2007). And a paper in the *Journal of the Science of Food and Agriculture* reported that organic potatoes are fairly consistently a richer sources of vitamin C than conventionally grown potatoes. Further, at least half of the studies analyzed found that other organically grown vegetables, especially leafy greens, had higher levels of vitamin C, and not a single study found lower levels of this vitamin in organic produce (Williamson 2007). Interestingly, the author still concludes that there is no reason to suggest that people switch to organically raised foods just yet. Of course, I respectfully disagree.

Organic produce also offers the benefit of not being contaminated with unhealthful substances such as pesticides. The same is true of animal products. Animals that are raised on unnatural or synthetic foods and dosed with antibiotics and hormones often aren't as healthy as animals that roam in the wild eating their natural foods. Some studies have found that fertility and weight declined in animals given conventional foods, while those raised on organic foods didn't suffer from such problems (Worthington 1998). In addition, chemical residues may remain in the tissues of conventionally raised animals, which are then ingested by the consumer. Plus, toxic substances from the environment, feed, and drugs can actually be concentrated in the flesh of animals in a process called bioaccumulation. One way to minimize your own toxic load is by only eating organic products, both plant and animal.

Obviously, most people don't fall over dead when they eat conventionally grown and commercial foods, so there is a lot of debate about whether organic foods are genuinely more healthful. In my opinion, that totally depends on the health and the immune system of the individual. People whose health is more compromised would be more sensitive to the toxins and other chemicals in conventionally raised foods. Admittedly, that would be hard to prove with the scientific method. We'd have to study many thousands of people over one or two generations to obtain meaningful results, and I venture that it would be almost impossible to find such a large group of compliant subjects, as well as the extensive funding for such a long-term study. Still, I believe that whenever we have the choice, the safest bet is to go for organically grown or raised, free-range, chemical-free, natural foods. At the very least, they taste better.

If you have the option available to you, it's also a good idea to buy local foods when possible. They're generally fresher and therefore more nutritious. Plus, small family farms and people who sell their produce at farmers' markets are generally more careful about how they grow things.

## Combating Poor Food Quality: Choose Only Fresh, Natural, Unrefined Foods

Fresh, natural, and unrefined foods are available in all markets as well as in many natural food stores. The key is to purchase foods that have to be prepared from scratch: whole grains, beans, fresh vegetables, fruits, nuts, seeds, organic eggs, fish, organic or free-range poultry, and so on. When purchasing prepared foods, look for those made from those same basic ingredients, things like whole grain breads, bean dishes, soups, salads, steamed and stir-fried vegetables, roasted whole organic chicken, and so on. It's best to avoid anything made with ingredients that are obviously not food, such as colorings, flavorings, dough conditioners, preservatives, and the like. I consider them "internal pollution." (I'll provide more guidance on prepared foods later in this chapter.)

It is heartening to find that people can actually enjoy changing their food habits to focus on fresh, natural, and unrefined foods—even children, who are so often viewed as disliking healthful foods. There is a growing movement to change the quality of foods in primary and secondary schools. Perhaps you'd think that's a wasted effort, children will demand their pizza and burgers and turn up their noses at Swiss chard. But here is a wonderful account, published in the *New York Times*, about what happened when the Promise Academy in Harlem introduced children to leafy greens: "Ebony, 12, had never seen Swiss chard until a month ago. She ate three helpings. 'I was like, "I don't want to eat that,"' she said of her first few months of meals at the Promise Academy. 'But I had to, because there was nothing else. Then it was like, "This is good."' Now she demands that her father, Darryl Richards, pick up chard at the makeshift farmers' market held once a month in the school cafeteria. They may even take one of the school's cooking classes together" (Severson 2005). From my own experience, eight of my students and I went to do a food demo in May 2008 at a public school in Harlem under the sponsorship of Touro College's Project Aspire. We showed sixty kindergartners a variety of fresh vegetables, both cooked and raw, and they gladly tasted beets, radishes, sweet potatoes, green beans, and other veggies, and took home recipes for their parents.

## Combating Poor Health: Prepare Your Food with Care and Attention

People who have problems with absorption and digestion need to cook their food well to make it more easily digestible. They may find raw vegetables and salads hard to digest because of the excessive roughage, in which case they'd be better off with soups and stews. Fruit is easily digested for some people, and too gas-producing or high in sugar for others. If you have digestive issues, you may need to work with a health care practitioner to determine the source of the problem; for example, you may have food allergies or intolerances and need to avoid or limit certain foods. Another approach is to keep a food diary. Record everything you eat, along with how you feel afterward. Perhaps you need to avoid certain vegetables or certain spices. Or you may discover that you're eating an awfully lot of a particular food, and that you can tolerate it better if you only eat it on occasion. If you take this approach, observe not just the foods you eat, but how they're cooked. Perhaps foods cooked in certain ways work better for you.

Whatever the source of your digestive difficulties, it will be beneficial for you to eat primarily home-cooked meals. This allows you to emphasize the foods and cooking methods that work best for you, rather than leaving it up to chance what will be available when you purchase prepared foods. Even if you can't eat three home-cooked meals each day, at least try for one or two. This is time invested in your own health and your family's health. In addition, getting sick is expensive, especially these days, so think of cooking healthful food as a good investment, in terms of both time and money.

## COOKING FROM SCRATCH

For the best of health, as well as for controlling what's in your meals, it's important to eat food cooked from scratch, rather than using mixes and packaged, canned, and frozen ingredients. These may be convenient, but they lack prana or qi, that indefinable life energy that replenishes us and gives us zest. Cooking from scratch and preparing delicious and healthy meals is creative and satisfying, too. Why deprive yourself of that pleasure?

There is much talk about the benefits of eating raw foods. That may be true for some foods, such as fruits, certain vegetables, and even very carefully selected seafoods, in the form of sashimi or sushi. However, many highly nutritious foods are hard to eat or digest if raw, such as grains and beans. And cooking makes many other foods easier to assimilate, especially in the case of plant foods, as it breaks down the proteins and cellulose walls and makes the nutrients more available to the digestive juices. For example, you absorb more beta-carotene from a cooked carrot than from a raw carrot. As described in the Nutrition Fact Sheet of the Feinberg School of Nutrition at Northwestern University, "The bioavailability of beta-carotene and other carotenoids increases several-fold during cooking because heat releases these substances from proteins to which they are bound in foods. The addition of oils or other fats to carrots, greens or other carotenoid-rich foods during cooking will optimize absorption" (Northwestern University 2007).

That said, I recognize that in today's busy world, cooking several meals a day may not be a viable option. One solution is to do a lot of cooking once a week, say, Sunday afternoons, making enough stock, soup, whole grains, and perhaps beans for four to five days. During the rest of the week you can add a piece of fish or some organic chicken plus a salad, and you've got dinner in about twenty minutes. Another solution is to compromise with some ingredients. Later in this chapter I'll offer some guidance on the healthiest convenience foods to incorporate into your cooking, as well as healthy options when eating out. If you continue to eat out or purchase prepared foods, be sure to read that part of the chapter closely, as it gives helpful tips on the most bone-healthy choices. Obviously, though, the best choices are restaurants or vendors that use high-quality ingredients and a "from-scratch" approach to cooking. If you do choose to continue using some packaged foods, read ingredients lists carefully and opt for products that don't contain any chemical additives, hydrogenated fats, sugars, fructose or high-fructose corn syrup, artificial colorings and flavorings, and so on. (And watch out for the new euphemism "evaporated cane juice," and even "organic evaporated cane juice," which is still sugar!) In other words, when you read the ingredient list, *if it doesn't sound like food, it ain't food.*

When planning a menu, aim to include the following elements in most lunches and dinners:

- A whole grain dish or something made with whole grain flour

- A source of protein, either beans or animal products (fish, chicken, eggs, meat)

- One or more green vegetables

- One or more red or orange vegetables

- A source of good-quality fats

That's the bare bones of it. If you want, you can even combine most of those essentials into a single one-pot dish, such as a soup or stew. As you can see from the list, dessert is optional. If you just can't live without it, restrict yourself to bananas, dates, or other fruits, or perhaps a small naturally sweetened cookie. For beverages, filtered or mineral water will do just fine.

# THE BEST FOODS FOR STRONG BONES

Let me make very clear what the best foods are for the bones—in this order:

1. Vegetables, *especially leafy greens*, and also roots and stalks (for the iron and calcium, and for vitamins K and C, which, together with protein, help deposit the collagen matrix)

2. Protein, such as animal foods, beans, and soy foods (for the collagen matrix)

3. Stock (for the minerals)

4. Whole grains (for the magnesium)

5. Foods rich in trace minerals, such as seaweeds, nuts, and seeds

6. Edible bones (for the calcium and other minerals)

7. Healthy fats (for the fat-soluble vitamins needed for the bones, such as vitamins K and D)

To underscore the approach of eating for bone health, the recipes in part 3 are generally arranged in the above order, although in most cases the fats are included in the recipes, not featured as a separate food. Every section, then, relates to bone health in a specific way. Let's take a closer look at these categories and review how each relates to bone health.

## Vegetables

Calcium, magnesium, potassium, iron, and other minerals are found abundantly in the vegetable kingdom, especially in produce that's organically grown. Of particular value for bone health are all the leafy green vegetables, such as kale, collard greens, mustard greens, arugula, bok choy, parsley, watercress, and mesclun, the only exceptions being spinach and Swiss chard, as explained below. Other vegetables especially helpful to the bones include broccoli, cabbage, carrots, zucchini, and acorn or butternut squash. In fact, the food that provides the most calcium *per calorie* is bok choy, at 790 mg per 100 calories when cooked. Other vegetables with a high calcium content include cooked mustard greens, with 495 mg calcium per 100 calories; raw celery, with 250 mg calcium per 100 calories; and steamed broccoli, with 164 mg calcium per 100 calories. For comparison, skim milk provides 351 mg of calcium per 100 calories, so the veggies are quite within the ballpark.

Some vegetables, most notably spinach and Swiss chard, contain a relative abundance of calcium but also contain oxalates, substances that may interfere with calcium absorption in some cases. However, people on low calcium diets (300 to 400 mg per day) are more efficient at overriding the effect of oxalates and absorbing calcium than people on diets high in calcium-rich dairy products.

## Protein Foods

As explained earlier, protein is essential for giving bones the flexibility that helps prevent fractures. There is controversy as to whether protein from animal or vegetable sources is better. For quite some time, the popular assumption was that a diet high in animal protein could contribute to osteoporosis. This assumption has been shown to be incorrect. Some people object to the consumption of animal foods for a variety of reasons. My viewpoint has always been that the choice to be vegetarian or not is a very personal one, and that either can be very healthful as long as the diet is balanced and the foods consumed are fresh, natural, and unrefined—and hopefully organic.

## Cooking with Stock

Cooking with stock is a very traditional way of increasing the nutritional value of dishes made with added liquid, such as soups, stews, grains, beans, and sauces. By cooking bones and vegetables for a long time over low heat, many of the minerals are leached out into the cooking water, making the stock highly nutritious and also alkalizing, especially if something sour has been added such as vinegar or wine.

## Whole Grains

In modern times, the primary grains that most cultures rely on for sustenance—rice and wheat—are usually stripped of their bran and germ and thereby made deficient in nutrients. Whole grains, such as brown rice, whole wheat, barley, oats, rye, millet, cornmeal, amaranth, quinoa, teff, and buckwheat, are excellent sources of complex carbohydrates, fiber, and B vitamins, and they're very satisfying to boot. Consuming sufficient amounts of whole grains (about a handful of cooked whole grain per meal) also means you need to consume less animal protein due to a concept known as protein sparing. When grains (or fats) provide more calories, this diminishes the body's need to metabolize proteins for energy. This conserves muscle tissue, and whatever is good for the muscles is good for the bones. In addition, whole grains are a good source of magnesium, which helps increase absorption of calcium from the blood into the bones.

## Foods Rich in Trace Minerals

Seaweeds, nuts, and seeds are some of the foods richest in trace minerals. As mentioned in chapter 3, trace minerals play an important role in bone health. Remember, less important than how much calcium you eat is the balance of minerals (and other nutrients). Eating foods rich in trace minerals will go a long way toward providing mineral balance.

Seaweeds, which are most commonly used in Japanese cuisine are rich in minerals, making them an excellent addition to healthful cooking. In fact, a study of osteoporosis in Taiwan found that those who include seaweed in their diet two or more times per week showed a slightly higher protection against osteoporosis (Shaw 1993). Seaweeds are also valuable for being especially high in iodine, which is necessary for good thyroid function. As discussed in chapter 3, the thyroid and parathyroid glands play an important role in bone health.

Nuts and seeds have the advantage of also being a great source of bone-healthy essential fatty acids, as well as plant protein. A handful of nuts or seeds a day is a good source of trace minerals, such as iron, boron, selenium, phosphorus, and magnesium.

## Edible Bones

Perhaps your initial response to the idea of eating bones is "what?!" But bones can be eaten when prepared in certain ways, and if you think about it, what better source of natural minerals for our bones than bones themselves? See the recipes in part 3.

## Healthy Fats

Good-quality fats are essential for bone health. As we apply the "three-bears-rule" again, too much is no good, but too little is no good, as well. You need to eat enough of these important nutrients, even if that means unlearning a fat phobia. The average postmenopausal woman needs about 65 grams of fat daily. That means you need approximately 2 or 3 tablespoons of good-quality fat per day in an eating regime based on vegetables, beans, grains, nuts, and seeds, or about 1 or 2 tablespoons if your diet also includes animal products. Nutritionist Udo Erasmus cautions against using any one type of fat exclusively because it won't contain a full profile of fatty acids and therefore might create an imbalance (Erasmus 1993). We need both omega-3 and omega-6 fatty acids. However, a diet high in polyunsaturated vegetable oils is skewed too much in favor of the latter.

# EATING OUT, ORDERING IN, AND CONVENIENCE FOODS

If you don't do your own cooking, you can still eat healthful meals that are mostly prepared from scratch. You can hire a private chef, perhaps to cook for you once or twice a week; you can buy high-quality prepared foods; or you can eat out in restaurants or order in. However, the more you choose the last three options, the less control you have over the quality of your food and the harder it is to use food to manage your health. But it can be done, and the rest of this chapter will show you how.

# Eating Out and Ordering In

People over fifty remember that breakfast and dinner, at least, used to be eaten at home in the company of one's family. In my own childhood, we ate all three meals at home. Only very rarely, once a month or so, did we go to a restaurant, and that was always an occasion for dressing up.

Since the latter part of the twentieth century, the situation has changed dramatically in the United States. In 1995, almost one-third of meals and snacks were consumed away from home, and close to 40 percent of meals and one-fourth of snacks eaten outside the house were from fast-food restaurants (McCrory et al. 2000). Close to half of family food dollars were spent outside the home. Six out of ten Americans ate at least one food product outside the home in the mid-1990s, whereas only four in ten did so in the mid-1970s (Nicklas et al. 2001). Another study found that in 1992 and 1993, nearly 40 percent of households in the United States ate breakfast out and that a majority of households buy lunch or dinner prepared outside the home in any given week (Jensen and Yen 1996). This isn't necessarily a bad thing. It just means we need to pay attention to the quality of the food we buy.

People don't cook much at home anymore for several reasons. Many feel they don't have the time, and others simply don't have the inclination. Perhaps the biggest factor is that so many women, who traditionally have done most of the cooking, now work outside the home and have little time for cooking (Freeman and Schettkat 2005).

Cooking from scratch, of course, remains the ideal, in terms of both nutrition and the energetics of how the food feels. There is something impersonal and disconnected about restaurant and prepared foods, no matter how fancy and elegant, whereas even very simple home-cooked meals have a nourishing feel to them that no restaurant can emulate. That said, I do believe that the quality of take-out food and restaurant food has improved considerably over the past ten years or so. I feel that you can now do reasonably well for your health with carefully chosen restaurant and prepared foods. And this is a good thing, since most people alternate between home-cooked meals, eating out, and ordering in, as shown by the statistics above.

For times when you need or want a little supplementary outside food that also helps your bones, here are some suggestions.

## CHOOSING YOUR SUPPLIER

Unless you live in a remote rural area, you probably have some nearby choices for purchasing prepared foods. Test the offerings of a variety of restaurants, coffee shops, and delis, including the prepared foods available in supermarkets, and pay careful attention to how the food feels to you. For example, I have four different markets within eight blocks of my house in New York City, and after tasting a variety of offerings from all, I find that only one of them consistently has tasty, good-quality prepared foods that I consider clean, even if it isn't usually organic. So that is where I normally purchase prepared foods if I need to. If you're lucky to have a natural food market near you, they may offer some prepared dishes made with organic or free-range products. Test their foods to see which ones work for you.

## CHOOSING YOUR DISHES

Just because you're eating out doesn't have to mean that your dietary principles go out the window. When ordering, try to approximate what makes for a healthful meal. General guidelines for the health of your bones include the following:

- Have a green salad at least once a day or, even better twice a day. The dressing should be simple, like olive oil and lemon juice. Don't choose fat-free dressing, as they contain too many strange ingredients.

- Have a good protein dish, such as fresh ocean fish, free-range chicken or meat. Choose organic or grass-fed whenever available. If you're vegetarian, or if you're just in a vegetarian mood, go for beans in soups or side dishes.

- Choose brothy soups such as chicken or fish soup, beef and barley soup, bean soups, and vegetable minestrone. Avoid tomato-based soups and cream soups, which often have a flour base.

- Include two or three cooked vegetables in every meal, in addition to the salad, such as cooked greens, beets, squash, zucchini, broccoli, green beans, bok choy, turnips, and so on. It's best to avoid frozen or canned vegetables, so find a place where the prepared vegetables are fresh, even if they aren't organic.

- Stay away from nightshade vegetables, including potato dishes and foods with tomato sauce, except maybe once a week.

- Avoid soft drinks and caffeinated drinks, including (and maybe especially) diet drinks.

- Stay away from commercial desserts made with sugar and flour, including cakes, cookies, pastries, pies, and, of course, ice cream. Buy your own fresh fruit for dessert or make your own from the recipes provided. This is better for your bones, your health in general, and your waistline, and it's easier on your pocketbook too.

## CHOOSING THE BEST OPTIONS IN VARIOUS RESTAURANTS

To round out the general guidelines above, here are some specific recommendations for the most bone-healthy options at various types of restaurants:

1. In coffee shops, you can get soups, salads, and protein dishes. Even though it's called a coffee shop, you don't have to drink coffee! Drink water or mineral water or have peppermint tea or another herbal tea. Avoid the desserts.

2. In Chinese restaurants, go for stir-fried vegetables (broccoli, green beans, snow peas, carrots, bok choy) with shrimp, chicken, tofu, or meat. Ask for brown rice instead of white, and request that MSG (monosodium glutamate) and sugar not be added to your food. They can usually do this for most dishes other than soups, as MSG and sugar are often added to the stir-fry dishes just before cooking. I must say I'm not so keen on Thai restaurants, as practically every dish and every sauce in those restaurants has sugar in it.

3. In Italian restaurants, have a salad and a fish dish or other meat dish, such as chicken piccata. It may seem heretical, but avoid pasta, or only eat a very small portion.

4. In more upscale restaurants, always get a good salad, fish or chicken, and cooked vegetables. I generally recommend picking a protein dish by its accompaniments. My personal preferences always to go polenta, greens, and mushrooms as side dishes. Avoid dessert, but if you can't resist, just steal a spoonful of someone else's chocolate mousse.

5. Mexican restaurants, where so many dishes are laden with cheese and chile peppers, may be a challenge. Meat or seafood dishes are probably your best choice, but try to avoid spicy entrées, which probably contain chile peppers. In terms of accompaniments, go heavy on the guacamole and light on the tomato salsas. Corn tortillas are preferable to flour, although with all the genetically engineered corn, that may now be a moot point.

6. In Japanese restaurants, miso soup and sushi or nori rolls are the best choices. Go easy on the tuna because of the mercury; better choices for sushi and nori rolls include whitefish, avocado, eel, and cucumber. Watch out for teriyaki; it's always full of sugar.

7. In Greek restaurants, good choices include salad, lamb dishes, as well as hummus and other appetizers. Some Greek restaurants have cut down on the olive oil, mostly to give the food a lower fat content. As a result, their dishes sometimes taste very sour from the lemon not balanced by the olive oil. Simply ask for a bottle and season your food with it as you like.

8. Indian restaurants have many nice vegetarian and lamb dishes. The food, however, is often spicy. You may want to ask for your dishes to be made very mild.

9. I don't trust fast-food restaurants nor do I like their food, and I encourage you to avoid them. According to John Andrews in his online article "Surprise Ingredients in Fast Foods" (2007), there are numerous toxic ingredients in the meat and even in the salad dressings, including MSG in almost everything. A salad à la carte may be the only healthy thing to eat at a fast-food place. But in most cases the side salads offered at the fast-food places are hardly a meal—and hardly what one would consider a real salad. And keep in mind that the meat on those salads probably isn't any higher in quality than the other meats they serve. Even seemingly simple items like rice can have ingredients like antifoaming agents. And unless you're lucky enough to live in New York City or Denmark, many of the offerings in a fast-food place are probably laden with trans fats.

## Convenience Foods

Although take-out and restaurant food may seem preferable in terms of time and convenience, you generally can't be certain of the ingredients or the quality of the food. And it can be expensive. There is a middle ground. You might consider purchasing certain convenience foods that can help you save time on cooking. Here are some ideas about healthful options. You may find other useful and convenient ingredients in your local markets. Just keep in mind that you want genuinely high-quality foods—devoid of chemical ingredients and as fresh, natural, and unrefined as possible.

### VEGETABLES

Sliced or chopped fresh vegetables, including onions, carrots, celery, zucchini, and mushrooms, are great for soups and stir-fries. They're as quick to use as frozen or canned vegetables, plus they taste much better and retain more of their nutrients. (Frozen or canned vegetables may lose as much as 20 to 80 percent of their nutrients in the processing, as well as their flavor.) For optimum nutrition and freshness, use them within a day or two.

Another great option is prewashed salad greens, which make it easy to eat your leafy greens daily. You may want to give them a quick rinse and spin them dry to refresh them and make sure they're pristine.

## PROTEIN FOODS

Rotisserie chicken, preferably organic or free-range, can make it a snap to put a bone-healthy meal together. For example, combine the chicken with some prewashed salad greens and brown rice (maybe left over from one of those Chinese meals), and you're set. Just don't forget to save the bones in a plastic bag in the freezer for making stock.

Even though I don't like most canned foods, I do use canned sardines in olive oil, good tuna in olive oil, and, in a pinch, canned salmon, as you'll see in the recipes. The sardines should *not* be skinless and boneless, as the bones are completely edible and valuable for their mineral content. Put canned sardines or tuna on a nice salad and add some lemon juice (you already have the olive oil the fish was packed in). Served with good whole grain bread, this makes for a nice lunch or light dinner.

For a snack or dip, ready-made hummus is a great protein dish. Just read the label carefully and avoid any made with processed or artificial ingredients. Use it as a dip for celery or carrot sticks (which you can buy precut), other vegetables, whole-grain pita chips, or organic corn chips.

## STOCKS

Making stocks from scratch, while easy, demands that someone be present in or around the kitchen for several hours. You could, of course, put the stock ingredients in a slow cooker and let them cook for a day. But if you really want to streamline, here are my recommendations on ready-made stock, which is an important source of minerals:

1.  Ready-made stocks may be available at your favorite market—fish, chicken, or meat stock, including demi-glace (a highly concentrated gelatinous veal stock that can be diluted). Usually they will be in the soup department.

2.  Organic vegetable and chicken stocks in aseptic cartons are quite good. There are several brands; try them all and pick the one you like best. But beware: at least one brand has sugar in it, or rather "organic evaporated cane juice." There is no need whatsoever to put sugar in a stock.

3.  Canned stocks, although I have not used them, are the next best choice, especially if organic. They may also be used to enrich other stocks.

4.  Don't use bouillon cubes or powdered stocks They are just seasoners, not high-mineral stocks, and they often contain MSG.

## MISCELLANEOUS

Some stores carry cooked polenta (a cornmeal mush) in sausagelike packaging. It keeps well until it's opened, and is delicious when pan-fried in butter or coconut oil, or sliced and grilled.

In terms of dessert, many stores carry organic unsweetened apple sauce with various other fruits, such as raspberries or strawberries. Get the small individual portions, they're great for dessert with a few sliced almonds. Another fun and easy dessert idea is stuffing pitted dates with a hazelnut or almond in the place of the pit.

This chapter has given you a great deal of information about how to cook and eat to maximize bone health. Our bodies are built of the foods we eat, so making changes to your diet can go a long way toward not just bone health, but overall health. Another major piece of the puzzle is movement. Just as our bodies were designed to function optimally on a diet of fresh, whole, natural foods, so to were they designed to move. In our increasingly sedentary culture, it can be a challenge to get enough exercise to maintain good health. Hopefully the information in the next chapter will give you the motivation to change if this is an issue for you.

# CHAPTER 7

# Movement and Exercise: An Important Part of the Program

*Morihei Ueshiba O'Sensei, regarded by many to be the greatest martial artist in modern times, deeply understood the larger flow of balancing. O'Sensei, the founder of the martial art of Aikido, was once asked by his students, "How do you keep your balance all the time?" The master laughed and said: "The art is not in trying to keep your balance, but in losing it and seeing how fast you can regain it. The reason you don't see me out of balance is because I regain it so quickly!"*

—Joel and Michelle Levey, *Living in Balance*

If you've heard it once, you've heard it a million times: Exercise is important for the bones. You've probably been told to walk, do weight training, and stretch so many minutes per day, so many times per week. Perhaps you are already doing this. It's a subject I don't get into much, as so many people are already talking about it that I feel it's been covered. But I had an experience while I was writing this book that made me think I should indeed talk about it—not to repeat what everyone has been saying, which you've probably already heard, but from my own idiosyncratic viewpoint.

If you were to ask me about my exercise regime, I would probably change the subject. I don't have one. Considering how much some people do, I'm embarrassed about that lack of commitment. I also know it's because of my very well-developed "mule response." Allow me to explain.

## THE MULE RESPONSE

When you pull a mule in one direction, the mule pulls with equal strength in the opposite direction. The harder you pull, the harder the resistance. From checking with my students, I've discovered this is a trait that most humans share, especially around the subjects of healthy eating and exercise. "Eat your peas!" "I'm not eating my peas." Have you ever been left at the table because you wouldn't eat your food? That certainly happened to me when I was little. And because of that mule response, which exhibited itself early on, I still didn't eat the whatever it was I didn't want to eat.

While I've obviously made huge strides when it comes to healthy eating, I'm still like that with exercise. "Do so many minutes per day of this or that!" Yeah, right. To tell the truth, exercise bores me. It feels all right, but not so great as to provide motivation to stick with a program. So I do stuff occasionally: a yoga class here, a Pilates class there, some stretching, some weights for a little bit. Then I forget for a week or two. Then I do it again for ten minutes. Then I'm off for two months. It's hardly a bone-healthy regime, but don't try to talk sense to me because my mule is very strong and always wins. Or that's how it used to be. But then things changed.

## THE SCHOOL OF HARD KNOCKS

Early in October 2005, my husband and I went to the movies. We sat in our usual third row from the back, in the middle. Then I decided I wanted some popcorn, so I got up to go fetch it. As I was going to the door, I realized I had my umbrella, so I stepped back to pass it to Bernie. In the very last row there was a space for a wheelchair, and I walked into it so as to reach over with the umbrella. What I didn't see was that there was a plastic child's booster seat on the floor—and it was a smooth floor for the wheelchair—so I stepped onto it with my right foot. As I was coming in with momentum, my foot and the booster seat slid forward, and I fell down into a split with my left leg bent at the knee and open to the side. As I slammed down to the floor I could feel something pulled around my left hip joint, and I thought, "Oh no! If I break a hip, I will never speak about healthy bones again. It would be too embarrassing." As I was a few months away from retirement age at the time (not that I was planning to retire from anything), no one would have been surprised if I had sustained a fracture.

To my good fortune and that of the movie house, it turned out I hadn't broken my hip (which usually means a break of the top of the femur). I had a small crack in the hip socket from the hard fall, which would heal on its own, and some badly sprained ligaments. This was very painful, but with a pair of crutches, lots of homeopathic remedies, and the help of some good acupuncturists, chiropractors, and an osteopath—and some patience—it eventually healed.

As I reviewed the fall in my mind, I became more and more convinced that if my bones had been weak, I would indeed have broken the top of my femur, given the angle at which I fell. And I asked myself what helped prevent this? What had I done—or not done—that kept me in one piece?

For me, the healthy food angle was sort of a given. I was very pleased that my healthy bone system had proven itself so clearly. Then I focused on my habits of movement. And I think I made some interesting realizations that I want to share with you, because they might be useful to you, as well.

# USE IT OR LOSE IT

We are told to exercise daily, or at least several times weekly. But how long do people keep up that kind of regime? A year, two, twenty? This approach does seem to work for a subset of people, and if you're one of them, congratulations! But there those of us who have no patience for this kind of regularity when it comes to exercise. As I contemplated why I hadn't broken my hip in that movie theater, I looked at what I had done over about forty-five years, since my early twenties. I had done a fair amount of gymnastics in my teens, as well as ballet and swimming, so I was pretty limber. After I came to the United States and got married, all that went by the wayside. For five years, I did very little exercise, as I considered myself active enough in routine, day-to-day tasks; besides we lived in a fifth-floor walk-up in New York City. You go up and down the stairs a few times with the baby and the groceries, and who needs extra exercise?

One day when the baby was about seven months old, I bent down to pick her up and my back gave way. I was stuck and couldn't get up or down. Finally I crawled into bed. My husband at the time, Rod, brought in an exercise specialist. I got a serious talking to. He showed me some exercises; my favorite was butt-walking (sitting and scooching forward one buttock at a time), which I think is a terrific way to strengthen your spine muscles. Soon enough my back improved. Vowing that it would never happen again, I tried to figure out how I could keep a strong back without spending too much time exercising. I settled on keeping my back flexible by bending down, nose to knees, for two minutes. This was something I could do even several times a day. And this is an exercise I continue to do *to this day*, although the body won't let the nose come too close to the knees anymore. But the hands still touch the floor.

Then I began to get into yoga, which was still pretty "far-out" back then, in the late sixties. I loved it. Sun salutations, dogs, cats, and all kinds of twists and bends came easy to me. Over the years I've done it off and on, at home or in classes, and lately with Pilates mat classes, always looking to keep my flexibility. One of the exercises I did with greatest pleasure, when I got around to it, was stretching the groin muscles by sitting cross-legged with the soles of my feet against each other and pushing my knees down toward the floor, or by bending one leg and placing the foot against the opposite thigh and leaning forward to touch the foot. In addition, I frequently sat in a cross-legged position with my knees very close to the floor (or the sofa if I was on the sofa). So my groin muscles were very flexible, and I strongly believe that this is what allowed me to stretch far enough (albeit a little further than I was used to) to keep me from breaking my hip.

Lately I've discovered a type of exercise that I really like. It's called NIA, for non-impact aerobics or "neuromuscular integrative action" (or, as my teacher says, "no inhibitions allowed"). My local gym has a NIA class for seniors that's basically dancing to music with attention to all of the muscle groups. It actually integrates dance, martial arts, and some yoga. This is great fun—and easy! I think I've finally found something I can continue, as it is more like dancing, which is fun, than "exercise," which feels so dutiful. Some of the people in the class have walkers or obviously painful bodies, yet even they can do a good number of the moves at their own pace.

# CREATING A PROGRAM THAT WORKS FOR YOU

So how does this apply to you? I genuinely believe that in order to create an effective exercise habit, you must think about what you can sustain not for weeks, but for decades. What sort of movement and exercise can you do that you'll enjoy and that won't elicit the mule response? What feels good to your body? In terms of bone health, three types of exercise are known to be helpful: weight-bearing exercise, strength training, and flexibility. As to the specifics, you have to choose forms of these types of exercise that are fun or sustainable for you and that incorporate as many of those details as possible.

## WEIGHT-BEARING EXERCISE

Weight-bearing exercise isn't as complicated as it may sound. It can be as simple as walking, hiking, dancing, or climbing stairs. Your own body weight will suffice; it isn't necessary to introduce additional weight. As mentioned in chapter 3, walking is excellent for bone health because it's the form of movement that most efficiently puts just enough gentle strain on the bones to promote their continued remodeling. Plus, it's something you can do almost anytime, anywhere, and there are no costs involved other than a minor investment of time, which will also be an investment in your health.

Walking just three to five miles a week can benefit your bones and your overall health—and it's likely to benefit you in other ways, too. You might find it meditative, or it may give you a chance to mull over issues that have been troubling you. Or you might walk with a friend and enjoy both exercise and social support. And if you do your walking outdoors in the sunlight, you'll be getting the vitamin D you need for strong bones, too.

## STRENGTH TRAINING

Another type of exercise that strengthens the bones is lifting light weights. This is something you can do at home, and a set of weights isn't very expensive. Especially considering how little investment is required, this activity can be very effective. A study of postmenopausal women at the Veteran's Administration Medical Center in Gainesville, Florida, found that weight training not only increased the strength of legs, arms, and shoulders, it also increased bone density by about 1.5 percent per year; the sedentary control group, on the other hand, lost about 2 percent annually (Thomas 1994). Over five or ten years, this could make a huge difference in the risk for fractures.

It isn't necessary to go to the gym to do weight training exercises, so don't let that stop you. Some years ago, one of my students decided it was time for an exercise program, but she didn't want to spend the money to join a health club, or even to buy dumbbells. So she started lifting kitchen chairs, gallon bottles with water in them, and other heavy household items. I saw her two months after she put herself on the program, and she was feeling and looking happier, peppier, and stronger.

Strength training takes other forms beyond weight-lifting. Any form of resistance will do, which is why it's also known as resistance training. Water exercise, isometric exercise, and using resistance bands all qualify here. The advantage to strength training is that it builds both muscle and bone. That building bone is advantageous for osteoporosis is obvious, but building muscle has benefits, too. For one thing, if you do take a fall, you'll have a better chance of recovering or catching yourself if your muscles are stronger. And additional muscle mass may provide some cushioning if you do hit the ground.

Swimming, while an excellent exercise, isn't really weight bearing because it is the water, not the bones, that bears the weight. Water exercise, on the other hand, does count for bone health, as it makes the body move against the resistance of the water. A study in Japan showed that water exercise, if consistently practiced, increases bone mineral density and encourages more general daily physical activity (Tsukahara et al. 1994).

## FLEXIBILITY

My own story of falling in the movie theater is a good example of why flexibility is so important for protecting the bones. Stretching, yoga, and tai chi are all excellent ways to promote flexibility and mobility of the joints. They're also beneficial because they promote breathing deeply, which indirectly protects the bones by reducing production of acids in the body. Yoga and tai chi are also excellent for balance, posture, and strength. As such, they can help prevent falls. Both are also generally gentle and easy, and therefore ideal for people of all ages. Tai chi, practiced daily in China, has been proven to reduce falls in the elderly (Li et al. 2005). You may find yoga to be the most satisfying exercise, as it just feels so good. Plus, it doesn't hurt the knees and is generally credited with stimulating all the endocrine glands and lowering blood pressure to boot.

## Cautions

Before you get started, a few cautions are in order. First, start slowly and gradually. If you're already active and want to increase your activity level further, a gradual approach is still best. If you injure yourself, you'll have to back off your exercise program or stop it altogether, at least for a while, and this will be a detriment to your bones. For those with weak bones, there are a few types of exercise to beware of. Steer clear of high-impact activities. It isn't necessary for you to run or do high-impact aerobics. Walking and water aerobics would be better choices.

# JUST GET MOVING

Ideally, you'd design an exercise program that combines walking or other weight-bearing exercise, strength training, and something for flexibility and balance, such as yoga or tai chi. As always, moderation is key. As mentioned in chapter 4, it is possible to do too much. For inveterate couch potatoes, getting some guidance for anything other than walking would be a good idea. If you already have fragile bones, do consult your physician before adopting a new exercise program. (The same is true if you have any other health conditions.) It may be a good idea to work with a physical therapist to develop a program appropriate for your current condition. Try the local Y, a gym, books, videos, or a personal trainer until you've developed a good program of healthful movement.

You may feel that you don't have time to exercise. That's a favorite excuse for many of us. But look at it this way (and I'll try to, as well): Thirty minutes or so three or four times a week seems to be enough to help keep the bones strong, and even fifteen minutes per day is good. That's just over 1 percent of your day, or 1.5 percent of your waking hours. Surely that's not too much time for something that has the potential to keep you strong, healthy, and fracture free into your old age. And if you should happen to break a bone at some point in the future, having a strong body will help you recover more quickly and avoid becoming immobilized.

Throughout this book, we've explored how to support bone health through physical approaches: primarily through diet, but also with movement. These approaches can go a long way toward promoting bone health, but an important aspect remains. Just as foods are most healthful when we look at them in their whole forms, so to must we consider the whole human being in order to achieve genuine healing. To that end, the next chapter offers some thoughts on the many nonphysical layers of our being.

CHAPTER 8

# The Spiritual Aspect:
# Strength from Within

*Thou knowest not what is the way of the spirit, nor how the bones do grow in the
womb of her that is with child.*

—Ecclesiastes 11:5

In this book we've spent a lot of time looking at very concrete aspects of existence: the
foods we eat, how we move, and the functioning of our bodies at a microscopic level.
We can fine-tune our lifestyle by eating lots of greens and mineral-rich foods and by
avoiding substances that drain minerals from our bones. We can adopt a carefully
crafted exercise regimen that enhances strength and flexibility and helps build bone.
Some of us may choose to take supplements or even pharmaceutical drugs. But will all
of that be enough to strengthen our bones? If, as I and many others believe, the body,
mind, and spirit are one, it may not be enough.

Human beings are complex and multilayered. For optimum health and well-being,
we must pay attention to our nonphysical, nonmaterial side—our spiritual side, if you
will. In this chapter we'll take a brief look at the metaphoric, emotional, and spiritual

aspects of our being so that you can consider whether any of these might be a factor in your bone health.

# DWELLING ON OUR WEAKNESSES

Our bones provide physical structure and keep us upright; metaphorically, they relate to our psychological and spiritual structure. If we look at the body as an expression of our inner selves, perhaps of how we think of ourselves, focusing only on one's faults could make this structure weaken over time.

When we are young, in our teens and early twenties, most of us feel invincible. Death will never get us. We can do anything. We know better how things should be done than all those older people who offer advice on the ways of the world. But as time goes on, we begin to find our limits, discover our weaknesses, and, eventually, feel that death is coming closer. Perhaps a weakness in our bones shows us our fear, our lack of connection with a core sense of self, of reality. Perhaps it shows us that we lack a support system we can fully rely on. Bones may weaken, according to Chinese medicine, not only from stress, but from fear.

Women are subject to fear because of the relentless social communication that tells us that we're not good enough. When young, we're not pretty enough, thin enough, sexy enough. When we get older, we're not sure we're good enough partners, mothers, or workers, and the judgments of our mates, other women, and society in general can all feed into this. As we get older and get to menopause, we're told that we're suffering from hormone deficiency, even though we're perfectly in tune with the natural order, which is set up to diminish our hormones. We think we're putting on too much weight, even though the natural order causes such weight gain for evolutionary reasons (to protect our bones!). We think we're getting too wrinkled and may regret that we're no longer seen as sex objects by most men (although we may in fact have happy and fulfilling sex lives). At this point in time, older women have no respectable place in our society, and all of these messages go to the deepest core of our self-esteem. Our mothers may have felt the same insecurities and passed them on to us. The end result is that we feel that unless we take the hormones, lose the weight, banish our wrinkles, try to look "sexy," and so on, we will utterly fail at being women. We fear that we've failed at aging gracefully any time we don't look younger than we are. What an impossible situation!

If we are living in this kind of fear, without good role models of strong older women and with a destroyed sense of self-value, if we are ignored or shunted aside by society, the media, even at times our children, we weaken and collapse figuratively. And so do our bones, literally. Therefore, it would be very helpful for each woman to find role models of an appropriate age that embody the values she would want to express herself. That way she knows what to aim for. I have decorated my walls with some photos of older women who look just gorgeous (without plastic surgery!). Find your own, and put them up as a reminder.

# REPRODUCING AND NURTURING

Throughout this book we've looked at our physical support structure, the skeleton, and how to keep it healthy. But what about other forms of support? All too often we receive only minimal support and must bolster ourselves simply by believing in ourselves against the odds. Since the dawn of humankind, our worth has been measured primarily by the allure of our bodies and the children we bear (two highly related factors!). What we are never told is that there are many ways in which women can "give birth"; children are one—and an important one—but our creations can also include art, books, businesses, and so much more. Likewise, there are many ways in which a woman can use her inborn instinct to nurture, supporting those close to her, such as friends, other people's children, coworkers, pets, and even casual acquaintances. We can also nurture our creations and ourselves.

By fully accepting our state, whatever it may be, and by seeing how we have brought ourselves to where we are through our choices—*and declaring those choices good and valid*—we can regain and boost our inner strength and structure. After all, everything is a lesson, and everything is connected.

# OUR SEVEN STRUCTURES

Let's take a look at our personal, emotional, and spiritual support systems, as they will hold up our physical structure—and not the other way around. What follows is my interpretation and synthesis of the work of many masters, principally the seven levels of judgment of George Ohsawa, founder of the macrobiotic diet and philosophy, and a philosophical view of the chakras from Caroline Myss, a pioneer in holistic health and the science of medical intuition. You may wonder how these wide-ranging philosophies relate to bones. Read on, and remember: As above, so below, and as is the inner, so is the outer. But does the body affect the mind, or is it the other way around? In body-mind relationships, all questions about causality are chicken-or-egg questions. I think we should consider this a two-way street: The body affects the mind, and the mind affects the body. To make changes, we can start at either end and get results.

1. **Physical: The body.** For a spiritual viewpoint on the body, I look to Rudolf Steiner, the German philosopher and founder of biodynamic agriculture, the Waldorf schools, and, most pertinent here, anthroposophy, a spiritual philosophy. Thomas Cowan, MD, a Concord, New Hampshire physician certified in anthroposophical medicine, wrote to me in a letter that, according to Steiner, "one's physical structure is the external manifestation and, in fact, the basis of an orderly thinking process and often an orderly society. Our bones are (or at least were) formed in precise mathematical relationships, which give our subconscious the experience of form, order, and logic." Thus, good bones give us a good basis for a coherent and orderly mental and emotional structure,

and weak bones will correlate with a lack of inner strength. This lack may have come through early neglect, abuse, or trauma. Recognizing this situation can be of help in motivating us to take care of strengthening our bones through diet and exercise. Then, as the bones get stronger, the other levels of our being will too.

2. **Tribal: Family, friends, and other relationships.** We need this structure for our sense of connection and belonging within a recognizable group of people who can give us support and receive ours in turn. If we have no mate or immediate family around, we need to create a structure of friends and coworkers that gives us that essential sense of tribal unity, without which loneliness can be truly unbearable.

3. **Emotional: Sense of self.** Knowing who we are in terms of that sense of "I am who I am" is a necessary inner structure that allows us to withstand the inevitable emotional blows that life sends our way. Any time we feel the need to ask, "Who am I?" we can assume that this sense of self, our emotional structure, is wobbly.

4. **Intellectual: Work, hobbies, and study.** Being gainfully employed or regularly occupied with satisfying activities is what we need to give structure to our days as well as our intellectual and creative energies. This isn't just about making a living, it's about being involved in something that helps us grow, as well as studying subjects that interest us. Having nothing to do, even if we are independently wealthy, is demoralizing and lowers our self-esteem, regardless of the thickness of our wallet.

5. **Social: Community and ecology.** We need to feel and understand that we are part of a larger community, part of this world, and that our actions impact our environment. Chaos theory, one of the more interesting models in the current sciences, states that everything is connected, and small disturbances in one area of the whole can create large and unexpected outcomes elsewhere: In other words, the beating of a butterfly's wings in Tokyo can eventually loosen a storm upon New York. We are part of the larger structure of our world, and we need to be conscious of that to find a larger meaning in our lives, to know that we matter in the universe.

6. **Philosophical: A view of life.** In my view, an essential component of our total structure is a philosophical understanding or model of how the world works. This helps us figure things out, make decisions, and predict what may happen if we follow one course over another. Religion provides this sort of view of life for a large majority of people. ("If you do this, then thus and such will happen"; for example, if you misbehave or don't follow the rules, you'll be punished.) Many of us also put together our own world view. I find that building a cohesive philosophical structure is one of the more fun activities in my life.

7. **Spiritual: A connection with the divine or the transcendental.** A feeling of awe tells us when we reach a connection with the divine. For our spiritual structure, we need to know that there is something unfathomable about the world we live in, that there

is always a mystery and an exquisite order far beyond our ken, and that we are a part of it.

Do you recognize an emptiness or lack in any of these seven structures in your life? If you often worry about your bones, look into these aspects of your existence as well. The first one, physical structure, is addressed throughout this book. The tribal, emotional, and intellectual structures can be addressed through a variety of therapies. Strengthening your social structure requires community activism, giving back, and volunteer work. To develop your philosophical and spiritual structure, look to introspection, meditation, and prayer. In addition, the five-element theory in traditional Chinese medicine says that excess worry is, like excess sweets, bad for the bones. Therefore, it is helpful to banish worry from your life as much as possible.

So, just as you increase your intake of vegetables to strengthen your bones and your overall health, consider attending to all of these issues to strengthen your overall inner stability. In other words, the foot bone's connected to the shin bone, the leg bone's connected to the hip bone, and all of the bones are connected to all the rest of the body. In the same way, the body's connected to the soul; it's all one package, and all of it deserves attention.

# CHAPTER 9

# Putting It All Together: It Is Possible to Regain Lost Bone

*Dem bones, dem bones gonna rise again.*

—Old spiritual

Hopefully this book has given you a great deal of food for thought and helped you see that it is within your power to promote the health of your bones. Part 3 of the book, Recipes for Healthy Bones, is really the core of the matter and will give you the practical tools for healthier bones.

Remember, simple everyday choices in regard to food, activity, and lifestyle can have enormous impacts on your health (or lack of it). In fact, it's precisely because these choices impact your body day in and day out that they have such profound effects. The principles in this book can help you retain bone health, and I'd go so far as to say that they may even be able to help you regain lost bone. As you'll see from the following case history, an integrated approach that combines diet, exercise, and even mental, emotional, and spiritual components can achieve remarkable results.

# CAN LOST BONE BE REGAINED? NINA'S STORY

Lost bone can indeed be regained, but it takes some work. If you doubt it, consider the case of Nina Merer, a New York City stress management consultant and licensed acupressurist who took some classes with me in the early 1980s. She was diagnosed with osteopenia in 1985, at the age of forty. Her condition was considered quite advanced, or "almost breakable." Initially, she tried prescribed calcium supplements, but finding herself with too many unpleasant side effects, such as intestinal bloating and headaches, she decided to go the "wholistic" route. Her doctor was doubtful, but supportive.

Why did she have such thin bones while she was still premenopausal? Basically, she had a number of risk factors: She was quite slim and Caucasian, she had no children, and her mother had osteoporosis. Nina also felt that hard work and hard play in her twenties and thirties had stressed and depleted her. She had an untreated thyroid condition, many digestive difficulties and food sensitivities, and a feeling of exhaustion. She also had felt an achy, arthritic pain, and a feeling as though her bones "were falling apart," which finally prompted her to seek professional help.

"It was a depressing diagnosis," she told me in 1997, "but it really served me. I began to think more deeply and decided to take responsibility, prevent further bone loss, and replace what I'd lost." After examining her lifestyle, she created a four-point program for herself that involved physical, mental, emotional, and spiritual components.

## 1. Physical

Nina's physical program included five elements: exercise, acupressure, herbs, dietary changes, and hormones.

Exercise. Having done moderate weight training for many years, Nina committed herself to a more systematic and intense program. She began running, and after becoming a marathoner, she eventually settled into running five miles about four times per week, a moderate distance in the runners' world. She also spent quite a bit of time stretching, as she always felt better when she did so.

Acupressure. Nina used various forms of daily self-help acupressure and got regular sessions from another practitioner to stimulate her body's energy points. She found it invaluable for both reducing stress and increasing energy.

Herbs. Working with a practitioner of Chinese herbal medicine, Nina started a regime of Chinese herbs to strengthen and tonify her system.

**Food.** Nina's well-rounded approach was twofold. She eliminated the calcium drainers (caffeine, nightshades, spinach, alcohol, and sugar, including fruit juices) and foods she had developed sensitivities to (wheat, oats, barley, rye, corn, dairy, eggs, red meat, vinegar, and fried and fermented foods). She focused on a healthy, whole foods, balanced diet, using organic foods whenever possible. Her meals consisted of gluten-free grains (buckwheat, rice, and millet), fish, organic chicken, some tofu, a little fruit, and, as she put it, "vegetables, vegetables, vegetables." Following the advice of her mother, Ella, every day she had one to three glasses of a mineral-rich blended vegetable drink made with romaine lettuce, carrots, parsley, radish, and celery. (You'll find a recipe for a variation on it, Green Drink, in part 3.)

As calcium enrichers, she regularly consumed seaweed and dark leafy greens and chewed on the bones of chicken and fish, eating the marrow when possible. She also consumed lots of toasted sesame seeds, as well as chia, sunflower, and fennel seeds. She got healthy fats in the form of borage oil supplements daily (helpful for the bones and to ameliorate arthritis), walnut or canola oil on her salads and sautéed vegetables, and soy oil, sesame oil, and the occasional avocado. (She'd always had trouble digesting fats, including olive oil, so for a long time she eliminated them from her diet; however, then she started feeling badly in new ways, with more arthritic pains, muscle pain, loss of muscle strength and size, unpleasant menopausal symptoms, and memory loss. When she reintroduced healthy fats into her regime, most of those complaints disappeared.)

**Hormones.** Upon entering perimenopause, Nina tried prescription birth control pills and then tried hormone replacement therapy with the standard drugs, but both made her feel "unacceptably uncomfortable," so she decided to change course. She read up on hormones extensively and asked many questions. Finally, in consultation with her gynecologist, she started taking specially compounded bioidentical hormones. Instead of taking them by mouth, she opened the capsules and put the oil on her skin, which worked well for her.

## 2. Mental

Nina realized that stress was a major problem in her life. To reduce it, she put her professional skills to work and designed a serious stress management program for herself, which later became the foundation of her professional work. In addition to the physical approaches of acupressure and exercise, her program includes affirmations, visualization, meditation, and breathing exercises. Her goal became to simplify and streamline her life, and get her priorities in order. All of this helped her become clear and focused, feel better, and, she says, "think straight, which was a major turning point."

## 3. Emotional

Nina found that the physical and mental aspects of her program were also beneficial emotionally. In addition, she used a system called reframing to learn to see obstacles as opportunities for learning. She found that another way to reduce her stress level was to focus on solving only solvable conflicts, instead of dwelling on things she could do nothing about.

## 4. Spiritual

Attending to her soul's needs, Nina found that meditation gave her deep satisfaction in new and profound ways. It helped her see the big picture for better clarity and planning, and helped her find creative solutions to her challenges.

## Nina's Remarkable Results

Nina's four-point program sounds like a serious, even radical, approach, doesn't it? Although it did involve some major changes to her lifestyle, the results were well worth it—and they astonished her doctor. After pursuing her program for twelve years, at age fifty-two and already well into menopause, Nina's wrist bone measured over the 100 percent level for her age group. Her spine bone density is a bit lower, and her hips are low normal, "fragile but not breakable." She estimates having gained at least 10 percent bone density, and now she is classified as mildly osteopenic. "If I hadn't done something I would have serious osteoporosis," she said. "It took a serious commitment, but I was willing to take a long time to correct a condition that took a lifetime to develop. This was a case of crisis-driven creativity. There are no quick fixes! Once you decide to take charge, it's doable."

# CREATING A PLAN THAT WORKS FOR YOU

We may not all need or want to embark on such an extensive regime, and some of us may not have the time. Fortunately, many of us aren't faced with a diagnosis as dire as Nina's was. Still, prevention is the best medicine. The program Nina developed for herself led to remarkable results and represents one ideal. Even so, it wouldn't necessarily be appropriate for everyone. The key is to look at yourself and your lifestyle, to take a close inventory of your diet and exercise habits, and to observe what works for you and what doesn't. Then, using the advice in this book, along with other resources and your own intuition about your body, you can begin to develop a program for bone health that's appropriate for you and your situation.

All of that said, I want to leave you with six main strategies to keep in mind for supporting or regaining your bone health and strength:

1. Avoid sugar and other refined sweeteners, white flour, hydrogenated fats, soft drinks, caffeine, and excessive amounts of nightshade vegetables, and don't pursue a low-fat or fat-free diet.

2. Go easy on the dairy products, and if you choose to use them, stick with organic products. Even if you're able to tolerate dairy products fairly well, still limit them to organic butter, plain organic whole yogurt, and unpasteurized cheeses, including Parmesan in small amounts on occasion.

3. Every day, eat some greens and vegetables, healthy fats, whole grains, nuts and seeds, and some good sources of protein such as animal products and beans.

4. Always cook with good-quality stock, preferably homemade, for its high mineral content.

5. Get some form of activity on a regular basis: Walk and lift things, stretch, or do formal exercise or weight training three or more times per week—or better yet, do all three!

6. Take a look at the rest of your life. You are the person best qualified to determine what may be missing, where you need help, and which aspects of your life need support and strengthening.

I hope this book has inspired you and given you the motivation to take charge of your bone health. Changes in diet and lifestyle can have profound effects, and you may prefer to give this approach a try rather than relying on pharmaceuticals that may do more harm than good. Brittle bones need not be an inevitable effect of aging! Explore the recipes in part 3 of this book to start on a delicious approach to bone health.

May your bones be good and strong the whole of your life so you can do the work and share the love and enjoyment that are your birthright.

# Recipes for Healthy Bones

*Food, not nutrients, is the fundamental unit of nutrition.*

—David R. Jacobs, Jr., Ph.D.

The following recipes were created to maximize their content of minerals, essential fatty acids, fiber, complex carbohydrates, and good-quality protein in order to support bone health. They aren't skewed for maximum calcium only. Rather, they offer well-rounded nutrition for healthy bones and are basically good for anyone's health. Some of the recipes include meat or other animal products, but there are plenty of choices suitable for vegetarians in the section on protein-rich dishes. Many of the recipes include suggestions about how or with what to serve them.

A few general notes: All grain and bean dishes, as well as soups, keep well in the refrigerator for 4 to 5 days. Dishes made with animal products are best eaten within 2 days.

As discussed earlier, organic ingredients are always preferable, especially when it comes to animal products such as poultry, eggs, meat, and dairy (if you choose to use it). The one exception is any fish labeled as organic. This means the fish was farm-raised; wild, sustainably harvested seafood is preferable. Free-range, organic, and grass-fed meats, poultry, and eggs are the very best choices if you have access to them. However, the available options won't always be perfect. If the choice is between commercial foods and nothing, choose whatever option is closest to fresh, natural, and unrefined, and eat it with gratitude!

Also, a quick note on cookware: What to cook is almost as important as what to cook it *in*. I cautioned against ingesting aluminum earlier, in the discussion of antacids. Aluminum cookware is also problematic, as it can taint the foods cooked in it with minuscule amounts of the metal, especially if the food contains acidic substances, such as vinegar, citrus juice, or tomatoes. The best cookware choices are porcelain, glass, enamel (as long as it's not chipped), stainless steel, and cast-iron for skillets.

# GLOSSARY OF INGREDIENTS

A few of the ingredients I call for may be unusual to you, so I've explained them below. In addition, I also offer guidelines on the healthiest choices for several more familiar ingredients. All of these ingredients can be found in natural food stores, Asian markets, or well-stocked supermarkets.

**Agar.** A flaked, colorless seaweed product, agar is used as a thickener for cold dishes, much like gelatin. It can also be added to stock in small amounts (about 1 tablespoon per 8 cups of stock), where it will provide substantial amounts of minerals. Although it may be available in Asian markets, it's probably best to obtain it at a natural food store, as the commercial variety is sometimes made with chemical softening agents, bleaches, and dyes.

**Cardamom.** A popular aromatic spice, cardamom consists of a white pod containing several black or dark brown seeds. The seeds have a strong taste. If you use the pods, they're easier to remove from the dish after cooking. (I don't recommend eating them.)

**Coconut oil.** Coconut oil is great to cook with, and because it contains so much saturated fat, it's more stable when heated. It's available in two forms, refined, which doesn't have any flavor, and unrefined, which tastes like coconut. I suggest using refined coconut oil for those few times when you want to fry something like French toast. Unrefined coconut oil is so delicious that it can be used unheated as an addition to food, much like butter.

**Flaxseed oil.** Flaxseed oil is high in polyunsaturated omega-3 fatty acids, but like other nut and seed oils it oxidizes very easily and can go rancid quickly. Keep it in the refrigerator or freezer, and use it mostly in salad dressings or as a topping for hot foods, including hot cereals. It's best not to heat flaxseed oil.

**Flaxseeds.** When recipes call for ground flaxseeds, you can purchase flaxseed meal for convenience. However, it's highly perishable and must be stored tightly sealed in the refrigerator or freezer. For optimum nutrition, grind the seeds yourself; a coffee grinder or spice grinder works well for this.

**Kombu.** Kombu, a key ingredient in Japanese stocks, is a seaweed that contains high levels of glutamic acid, a natural flavor enhancer, as well as a variety of minerals. When cooked with beans, it enhances their digestibility.

**Miso.** This traditional fermented soybean paste is rich in beneficial, gut-healthy bacteria. It's best not to boil it, so as to keep those bacteria active. For the same reason, choose unpasteurized forms and store miso in the refrigerator. It won't "go bad" at room temperature (it's bad already, meaning fermented), but storing it in the fridge will ensure it keeps maturing slowly.

**Sea salt.** These recipes call for sea salt. In contrast to commercial salt, it has a higher mineral content and is free of chemical additives, such as agents to keep it flowing freely. If you use commercial salt, kosher is probably the best bet, as it's unlikely to have added ingredients. *Fleur du sel* and other specialty sea salts are wonderful for use at the table.

**Sesame oil.** Like most seeds, sesame seeds are rich in healthful polyunsaturated oils. There are three kinds of sesame oil: Unrefined is pressed and filtered, has nothing added, and has a clearly distinguishable sesame taste. Refined, which is bleached and deodorized, lacks flavor, and I don't recommend it. Toasted sesame oil is made from seeds that have been toasted at high heat. It has a strong flavor and shouldn't be used for cooking, as it has a lower smoke point and shouldn't be reheated. Use it only as a flavoring after cooking, such as on stir-fried dishes or steamed vegetables.

**Tamari and shoyu.** These two different kinds of brewed soy sauce taste similar but are made slightly differently. Tamari is made with soybeans, salt, and a culturing agent. Shoyu is made with the same ingredients plus wheat, so those who are sensitive to wheat might want to avoid it. The best-quality soy sauces are brewed for about 18 months; look for them in natural food stores. Some commercial varieties have flavorings and other additives and may be made in as little as 3 days. I recommend using traditionally brewed varieties, even though they're more expensive.

**Umeboshi vinegar.** This Japanese product is extremely useful for seasoning soups, stews, dressings, dips, and spreads. It isn't actually vinegar at all, but rather a by-product of the manufacture of umeboshi plums, which are plums pickled in brine; a close equivalent would be sauerkraut juice. Umeboshi vinegar is both salty and sour and imparts a light and delightful touch to otherwise dense or heavy foods. It is alkaline, as opposed to conventional vinegar, which is highly acidic. If you can't find it, replace 1 teaspoon umeboshi vinegar with ½ teaspoon lemon juice mixed with ½ teaspoon water and ⅛ teaspoon sea salt.

**Water.** As discussed in chapter 3, clean, filtered, artesian water or spring water is always preferable to chlorinated and fluoridated tap water. Of all the contaminants that might be present in drinking water, I consider fluoride the most objectionable for bone health, as it has been found to increase the brittleness of bones. So make sure the water you consume, even the water you use for cooking, is free of fluoride. If you purchase a filter, make sure it removes fluoride as well as other contaminants.

# VEGETABLE RECIPES

For an optimum intake of minerals, include in your diet five to seven servings daily of a variety of vegetables:

- Dark leafy greens, both cooked and raw, such as kale, collard greens, mustard greens, turnip greens, watercress, arugula, chicory, escarole, mesclun, mixed baby greens, fresh chopped parsley, and the like (with the exception of spinach and chard)

- Squashes and root vegetables, including carrots, parsnips, yams, turnips, and rutabagas

- Cruciferous vegetables (such as broccoli, cabbage, cauliflower, and Brussels sprouts), and, in truth, all other vegetables, including onions, celery, garlic, ginger, radishes, and scallions, with the possible exception of nightshade vegetables (tomatoes, potatoes, eggplants, and peppers)

I can't overstate the importance of eating your vegetables, especially greens. They really must be part of any healthful eating style. In addition to calcium, leafy greens are also rich in other nutrients, such as iron, vitamin A, and vitamin K, which is so important for bone health due to its role in the formation of the collagen matrix. In his book *Diet and Nutrition* (1978), Rudolph Ballentine, MD, has put forward one theory as to why so many people now ignore these important foods: The modern preparation method of steaming instead of boiling generally yields tough and bitter greens. Strong-tasting greens should always be boiled for 15 to 20 minutes, uncovered, in plain unsalted water, and then drained and prepared as desired for the dish. The boiling removes the bitter tastes and makes the greens softer and sweeter. Even when cooked this way, dark leafy greens are high in nutrients. For example, just 1 cup of boiled collard greens contains about 80 percent of the recommended daily intake of vitamin A, 20 percent of the vitamin C, 15 percent of the calcium, and 8 to 10 percent of the iron (Kirschmann and Kirschmann 1996).

## Leafy Greens

## BASIC GARLIC GREENS

*Dark green leafy vegetables should be consumed almost daily for healthy bones, and this dish makes it easy and appetizing to do so. It's great as a side dish for lunch or dinner, and if you're willing to try something different, you'll also find it's a tasty accompaniment to a hot, savory breakfast cereal. Another great way to incorporate greens into breakfast is to combine them with eggs for a "green scramble." For a version really packed with calcium and other minerals, check out the next recipe.*

½ pound kale, collard greens, or mustard greens

1 teaspoon extra-virgin olive oil

2 cloves garlic, chopped

1 to 1½ cups chicken stock (pages 183 and 184), vegetable stock (pages 181 and 182), or water

Pinch of sea salt

Pinch of freshly grated nutmeg

1. Remove the tough stems from the greens. (One easy way to do this is to fold each leaf in half and slice out the stem.) Wash the leaves well and pat dry. Stack the leaves atop one another, then cut them lengthwise and then crosswise to end up with bite-size pieces.

2. Heat the oil in a large saucepan over medium-high heat. Add the garlic, stir for 1 minute, then add the greens and the stock and push the greens under the liquid with a wooden spoon. Simmer, uncovered, for about 15 to 20 minutes, until the greens are tender. Add the salt, grate a dusting of nutmeg over the greens, and cook and stir for 2 more minutes before serving.

Makes about 4 servings.

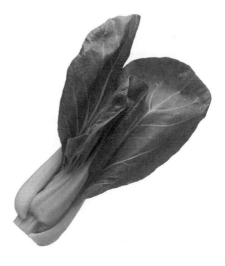

# PRESSURE-COOKED SOUTHERN COLLARD GREENS

*Thanks to Altheada Johnson for the inspiration for this recipe! Collard greens are a traditional side dish in the South, where they're always made with some salted meat, such as a ham hock or smoked turkey leg. Interestingly, these ingredients also contain bones, and the dish itself usually includes some vinegar. The upshot is that because the vinegar draws some calcium from the bone (and because collard greens are high in minerals), this dish is a fine source of absorbable minerals, including calcium. For that same reason, it's important to omit the vinegar if you make a vegetarian or bone-free version. This is a great dish to serve with rice and beans, especially black-eyed peas for New Year's Day. You can also make this recipe in a regular saucepan, in which case you should cook the meat for 1 hour and simmer the greens for about 30 minutes. Everything else is the same.*

    1 ham hock, or a piece of smoked turkey with bone

    2 cups chicken stock (pages 183 and 184) or water

    1 tablespoon wine vinegar or apple cider vinegar

    2 bunches fresh collard greens

    1 medium yellow onion, chopped

    3 cloves garlic, minced

    ½ teaspoon freshly ground pepper

    4 scallions, thinly sliced, for garnish (optional)

1.  Combine the ham hock, stock, and vinegar in a pressure cooker and cover securely. Bring up to pressure, then lower the heat to maintain pressure and cook for about 30 to 40 minutes. Allow the pressure to come down naturally, then remove the meat from the bone and set it aside. Discard the bone and leave the liquid in the pot.

2.  While the meat is simmering, prepare the greens. Remove the tough stems (one easy way to do this is to fold each leaf in half and slice out the stem), then wash the leaves well and pat dry. Stack the leaves atop one another, then cut them lengthwise and then crosswise to end up with bite-size pieces about 2 inches square.

3.  Add the chopped greens, along with the onion, garlic, and pepper, to the liquid in the pressure cooker. Cover securely, bring up to pressure, then lower the heat to maintain pressure and cook for 10 minutes. Bring the pressure down quickly by placing the pressure cooker in a basin of cool water.

4.  Add the meat to the greens and reheat briefly. Garnish with the scallions and serve piping hot.

    Makes 4 to 5 servings.

# SPICED KALE WITH CARROTS AND TURNIP

*For this recipe, you can prepare the spice blend ahead of time. It will keep well in a dry, tightly capped glass jar and makes a tasty addition to other dishes. You can make this recipe with turnip greens or collard greens, as well.*

Seasoning Blend
  2 teaspoons dried oregano
  2 teaspoons dried thyme
  1 teaspoon freshly ground black pepper
  1 teaspoon freshly ground white pepper
  1 teaspoon garlic powder

  1 tablespoon extra-virgin olive oil
  1 medium onion, diced large
  1 to 3 teaspoons Seasoning Blend
  3 small carrots, cut into matchsticks
  1 medium turnip, diced large
  2 cups vegetable stock (pages 181 and 182)
  ½ teaspoon sea salt
  1 bunch kale

1. Prepare the spice blend by mixing the oregano, thyme, black and white pepper and garlic powder until thoroughly combined.

2. Heat the oil in a large saucepan over medium heat, then add the onion and sauté for about 2 minutes, until translucent. Add the spice blend to taste (1 teaspoon is mild, 3 is strong) and stir for another minute or two.

3. Add the carrots and turnip and sauté for about 4 to 5 minutes, then add the stock and salt. Stir well to pick up all browned bits from the bottom of the pot. Lower the heat, cover, and simmer for 20 minutes.

4. Meanwhile, prepare the greens. Remove the tough stems (one easy way to do this is to fold each leaf in half and slice out the stem), then wash the leaves well and pat dry. Stack the leaves atop one another, then cut them lengthwise and then crosswise to end up with bite-size pieces about 2 inches square. Add them to the saucepan, pushing them under the liquid and turning the vegetables. As the kale begins to cook, it will shrink and soften. Simmer 15 minutes longer, uncovered, stirring once or twice. Serve hot as a side dish.

Makes 4 to 6 servings.

# STIR-FRIED BOK CHOY WITH SHRIMP

*For a vegetarian variation, replace the shrimp with cubed seasoned, smoked tofu (available at natural food stores). If you use shrimp, keep the shells for stock; just throw them in a bag in the freezer until you're ready to use them.*

> 4 leaves bok choy
>
> 1 tablespoon extra-virgin olive oil
>
> 2 large cloves garlic, minced
>
> ½ teaspoon minced ginger
>
> 2 scallions, thinly sliced
>
> 2 tablespoons vegetable stock (pages 181 and 182) or water
>
> 2 tablespoons natural soy sauce (shoyu or tamari)
>
> 12 medium shrimp, peeled and deveined

1. Wash the bok choy leaves well. Cut off and discard the bottom 1 inch, then cut off the greens along the thick white stem. Cut the stems in half lengthwise, then slice crosswise into ½-inch pieces. Pile up the greens, give them two cuts lengthwise, then cut them crosswise into 1- to 2-inch pieces.

2. Heat a wok or large sauté pan over medium-high heat, pour in the oil, and then, after a few seconds, add the garlic, ginger, and scallions. Stir or toss for about 30 seconds, then add the bok choy stalks and stir for another 1 to 2 minutes. Add the stock and 1 tablespoon of the soy sauce, then turn down the heat to low, cover, and cook for about 6 to 8 minutes.

3. Raise the heat to medium-high, add the bok choy greens, and stir for 1 to 2 minutes, until they're wilted. Add the shrimp and sprinkle with the remaining tablespoon of soy sauce. Stir for 2 to 4 minutes, until the shrimp firms, curls up, and becomes reddish pink. Serve immediately.

Makes 2 to 3 servings.

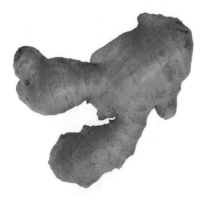

# BROCCOLI RABE WITH ROASTED GARLIC AND RED BELL PEPPER

*This dish can take the place of salad. After simmering the broccoli rabe, you can drink a cup of the "pot likker," or what my children used to call "greens water," with a dash of lemon juice or umeboshi vinegar for an excellent mineral-rich tonic. However, don't keep this cooking water for drinking or cooking with later, as it turns very bitter once it cools.*

1 head of garlic, cloves separated but unpeeled

1 teaspoon plus 1 tablespoon extra-virgin olive oil

1 bunch broccoli rabe (about 1 pound)

4 cups vegetable stock (pages 181 and 182) or water

1 large red bell pepper

1 tablespoon flaxseed oil

1 tablespoon freshly squeezed lemon juice

1. Preheat the oven to 400°F. Rub the garlic cloves with the 1 teaspoon olive oil, place on a baking sheet, and roast for 20 to 25 minutes, until soft but not burned. Peel and set aside.

2. Meanwhile, prepare broccoli rabe. Cut off the tough stems, wash the leaves and broccoli-like buds well, then coarsely chop into bite-size pieces.

3. Bring the stock to a boil in a medium saucepan, add the broccoli rabe, and lower the heat to maintain a simmer. Put a plate on top of the broccoli rabe to keep it submerged and cook for about 15 to 20 minutes, until tender. Drain the broccoli rabe.

4. Roast the red pepper by placing it directly over a gas flame and turning it with tongs until it is black and charred all over. Alternately, roast the pepper under the broiler or in a 400°F oven, also turning until blackened all over. Place the charred pepper in a small pot and cover or enclose it in a brown paper bag to let it sweat and loosen the skin. After 20 minutes, wash the pepper under running water to get all of the charred skin off. Discard the stem and seeds, then cut lengthwise into strips and across into squares.

5. Combine the 1 tablespoon olive oil, the flaxseed oil, and the lemon juice, and mix thoroughly. Toss the broccoli rabe with the garlic, bell pepper, and olive oil mixture. Serve at room temperature.

Makes about 4 servings.

# CURRIED BROCCOLI RABE WITH PARMESAN CHEESE

*This delicious dish is a combination of Indian and Italian ideas. It may sound unusual, but it comes together quite nicely. You can also make this with mustard greens in place of the broccoli rabe.*

    1 bunch broccoli rabe (about 1 pound)

    2 cups water

    2 tablespoons clarified butter (page 228) or extra-virgin olive oil

    3 large cloves garlic, thinly sliced

    1 tablespoon curry powder

    ¼ cup grated Parmesan cheese

1. Trim away the tough stems of the broccoli rabe and wash well.

2. Meanwhile, bring the water to a boil in a large saucepan. Add the broccoli rabe, lower the heat to maintain a strong simmer, and cook for about 10 minutes, until bright green and tender. Remove from the pot and chop into bite-size pieces. Discard the cooking water.

3. Heat the butter in a large skillet over medium heat, add the garlic, and sauté for 2 to 3 minutes, until lightly browned. Add the curry powder and stir well for 1 minute. (The curry powder will foam up; this is fine.) Add the broccoli rabe and continue to sauté for about 5 to 8 minutes, stirring often.

4. Sprinkle in the Parmesan, mix thoroughly, and serve.

Makes about 4 servings.

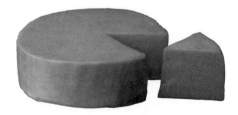

# GINGERED KALE WITH MISO-BROILED TOFU

*This is a flexible recipe. You can make both elements and serve them together, or you can make just the greens, as a side dish, or just the tofu, which makes a nice snack or appetizer. You can also substitute mustard greens or collard greens for the kale. The water left over from cooking the greens is nutritive, and delicious if you add a bit of lemon juice or umeboshi vinegar; try drinking a cup of it while you cook the rest of your meal.*

Miso-Broiled Tofu

> 12 ounces firm tofu
>
> 1 tablespoon mellow barley miso
>
> 1 teaspoon freshly squeezed lemon juice
>
> ½ teaspoon prepared mustard
>
> 1½ teaspoons extra-virgin olive oil
>
> 1 tablespoon water

Gingered Kale

> 1 large bunch kale, tough stems removed
>
> 3 cups water
>
> 8 thin slices of ginger
>
> 1 tablespoon extra-virgin olive oil

1. To prepare the tofu, oil a shallow baking pan, then slice the tofu into eight ½-inch thick slabs and arrange them in a single layer in the pan.

2. Combine the miso, lemon juice, mustard, oil, and water in a small bowl and mix with a fork until they form a thickish paste. Brush or smear the paste over both sides of the tofu slices and let stand for 15 to 20 minutes. Preheat the broiler.

3. Broil the tofu for about 5 minutes on each side, until nicely browned. Cut the broiled tofu into large pieces, cutting each slice once lengthwise and twice cross-wise, and set aside.

4. While the tofu is marinating, prepare the kale. Remove the tough stems from the kale (one easy way to do this is to fold each leaf in half and slice out the stem), then wash the leaves well and pat dry. Bring the water to a boil in a soup pot over high heat, then add the kale and 4 slices of the ginger. Lower the heat and simmer, uncovered, for about 15 minutes, until tender, pushing the greens under the water from time to time with a wooden spoon.

5. Fish out the greens and transfer to a colander to drain, discarding the ginger. Chop coarsely and set aside. Mince the remaining 4 slices of ginger.

6. Heat the oil in a large skillet over medium-high heat, add the minced ginger, and sauté for 30 seconds. Add the tofu, then add the chopped greens. Stir gently and cook a few minutes longer, until heated through. Serve hot.

Makes 4 servings.

# MIXED GREEN SALAD

*This standard salad is always pleasing and goes with everything. Feel free to vary the greens or add other ingredients.*

4 cups mixed baby greens or mesclun, loosely packed

1 tablespoon extra-virgin olive oil

1 tablespoon flaxseed oil

1 tablespoon freshly squeezed lemon juice

1 teaspoon umeboshi vinegar (see page 145)

1 teaspoon mustard

1 Belgian endive, sliced crosswise ½ inch thick

1. Place the greens in a serving bowl.

2. Combine the olive oil, flaxseed oil, lemon juice, umeboshi vinegar, and mustard in a small bowl or jar, and whisk or shake until thoroughly combined. Pour the dressing over the greens and toss well.

3. Divide the salad onto individual plates, and sprinkle the Belgian endive slices over each portion.

Makes 4 servings.

## Roots and Squashes

### BAKED BUTTERCUP SQUASH

*Many people consider buttercup squash (a squat, green winter squash) to be the most delectable winter squash. However, this cooking technique can be used with any hard winter squash or pumpkin. The only thing that might vary is the cooking time. Any leftovers make a delicious soup; just blend them together with sautéed onions and stock.*

> 1 medium buttercup squash
>
> 2 tablespoons stock, or as needed
>
> 1 to 2 tablespoons butter, flaxseed oil, or extra-virgin olive oil

1. Preheat the oven to 400°F and line a baking sheet or baking pan with parchment paper.

2. Scrub the squash well, cut them in half from stem to end, leaving the seeds in place, and brush the cut edges with a little olive oil. Place the squash halves cut side down on the prepared baking sheet and bake for about 1 to 1½ hours, depending on the size. The squash is done when a knife goes through the flesh easily.

3. Remove the seeds with a spoon and discard. Mash the squash in the skin, moistening the pulp with a little stock and adding butter, flaxseed oil, or olive oil to taste. Spoon onto individual plates as a side dish.

Makes about 4 servings.

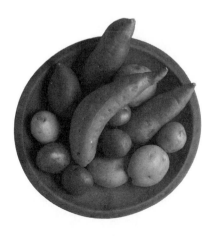

# BUTTERNUT SQUASH WITH ONIONS AND TARRAGON

*This is a delicious and easy way to prepare squash. If you have any leftovers, they make a great soup. Just puree them in a blender with enough stock or water to reach the consistency of a creamy soup, then heat and season to taste with salt and pepper.*

> 1 tablespoon extra-virgin olive oil
>
> 1 cup chopped onion (about 1 large yellow onion)
>
> ½ teaspoon dried tarragon
>
> 1 medium butternut squash, peeled and diced large
>
> ½ teaspoon sea salt
>
> Vegetable stock (pages 181 and 182), chicken stock (pages 183 and 184), or water

1. Heat the oil in a large saucepan over medium-high heat, then add the onion and sauté for about 2 minutes, until translucent.

2. Stir in the tarragon, then add the squash, sprinkle the salt over the top, and mix well. Add stock to a depth of ½ inch, then cover and cook over very low heat for about 25 to 30 minutes, until the squash is soft. Serve hot.

Makes 4 servings.

# YAM PUREE

*Here is an excellent way to get beta-carotene and essential fatty acids into people who dislike healthy foods. The unrefined coconut oil adds a delicious taste. Most of the tubers sold as "yams" are actually sweet potatoes; true yams are similar to sweet potatoes but grow primarily in tropical areas and are seldom sold in the United States. However they're labeled, choose varieties with a deep orange color, as they're sweeter, more moist, and higher in beta-carotene.*

> 2 medium sweet potatoes or "yams"
>
> Vegetable stock (pages 181 and 182)
>
> 1 teaspoon flaxseed oil
>
> 2 teaspoons unrefined coconut oil

1. Peel the sweet potatoes and cut them into big chunks. Place them in a medium saucepan and add enough stock to come up about ½ inch from the bottom. Bring to a boil over high heat, then lower the heat, cover, and simmer for about 30 minutes, until soft. Strain and reserve the stock.

2. Mash the sweet potatoes with a fork or a potato masher, using enough of the reserved stock (about ½ to 1 cup) to attain the consistency you like. Then add the flaxseed oil and coconut oil and mix well. Serve hot.

Makes about 6 servings.

# GRATIN OF ROOT VEGETABLES

*This is a nice warming vegetable dish for cold weather. Roots are a fine source of minerals, including calcium, iron, and potassium. For a great vegetarian meal, serve this over polenta, brown rice, or whole wheat couscous, accompanied by lentil soup and a salad.*

1 small rutabaga, peeled, halved lengthwise, and sliced ½ inch thick

1 sweet potato or yam, peeled and sliced ½ inch thick

2 small turnips, peeled and sliced ½ inch thick

1 medium parsnip, peeled, and sliced ½ inch thick

2 tablespoons extra-virgin olive oil

2 tablespoons whole wheat pastry flour

⅔ cup hot vegetable stock (pages 181 and 182) or vegetable blanching water

½ teaspoon sea salt

Freshly ground black pepper

¼ cup toasted whole wheat bread crumbs

1. Bring about 6 cups of water to a boil in a soup pot over high heat, add the rutabaga, and blanch for 5 minutes. Add the sweet potato, turnips, and parsnip and blanch for another 5 minutes. Drain the vegetables, reserving the water if you'd like to use it in place of the vegetable stock.

2. Preheat the oven to 400°F. Oil an ovenproof casserole, then place the vegetables in the casserole, overlapping the slices.

3. Heat the oil in a small saucepan over medium heat, then add the flour, stirring continuously for about 3 to 5 minutes, until fragrant and lightly browned. Whisk in the hot stock (or ⅔ cup of the reserved blanching water), stirring vigorously with the whisk first, then with a wooden spoon, until the mixture thickens and is lump free. Bring to a boil, stirring all the while. Add the salt, turn down the heat as low as it will go, cover, and cook at a low simmer for about 10 minutes, stirring on occasion. Add pepper to taste, along with more salt if needed.

4. Pour the sauce over the vegetables, cover, and bake for about 35 minutes. Uncover, sprinkle with bread crumbs, and bake about 25 minutes longer, until all of the vegetables are tender.

Makes 6 servings.

# BRAISED FENNEL

*Surprisingly tasty, this works well as a side dish for fish, chicken, pasta, or a bean casserole. It's especially important to choose organic citrus whenever you're using the zest, to avoid any chemical residues on the peel.*

1 bulb fennel

3 tablespoons extra-virgin olive oil

½ cup chicken stock (pages 183 and 184) or vegetable stock (pages 181 and 182)

Grated zest of ½ lemon

2 tablespoons freshly squeezed lemon juice

½ teaspoon sea salt

Freshly ground pepper

1. Cut the stalks off the fennel. Chop some of the feathery greens well, to yield about 1 tablespoon, and discard the remainder of the stalks. Cut the fennel bulb in half vertically, through the root, then vertically once again, into quarters. Trim away the core and dice the fennel.

2. Heat the oil in a large skillet over medium heat and add as much fennel as will fit in a single layer. Cook without stirring for 3 to 4 minutes, until the edges begin to brown. Flip the fennel over and cook the other side for another 2 to 3 minutes. If need be, transfer to a separate bowl and repeat with the rest of the fennel.

3. Return all of the fennel to the skillet and add the stock, lemon zest and juice, and salt. Bring to a boil, then lower the heat, cover, and simmer for about 10 to 12 minutes, until soft. Serve hot, with a grinding of black pepper on top.

   Makes 3 to 4 servings.

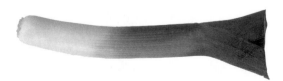

# Other Vegetables

## BROCCOLI WITH MUSHROOMS

*Here is a delicious and simple way to prepare this popular vegetable.*

2 stalks broccoli

1 tablespoon extra-virgin olive oil or coconut oil

2 large cloves garlic, minced

4 ounces mushrooms, sliced

¼ teaspoon sea salt

¼ cup water

Toasted sesame oil (optional)

1.  Cut the florets off the broccoli stalks and set aside. Cut away the tough lower end of the stalks, then peel the stalks with a vegetable peeler or sharp knife. Slice the stalks thinly on the diagonal and set aside.

2.  Heat the olive oil in a large skillet or wok over medium heat, then add the garlic and sauté for 10 seconds. Add the mushrooms and sprinkle with the salt. Stir and shake for about 3 minutes, until the mushrooms begin to release some of their liquid. Add the broccoli stems and mix well. Cover, turn down the heat to low, and cook for 5 minutes.

3.  Add the broccoli florets, mix thoroughly, then add the water, cover, and cook for 5 to 6 minutes, until the florets are a deep green. Serve immediately, sprinkled with the sesame oil if you like.

    Makes 4 to 6 servings.

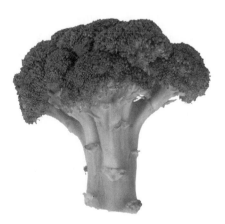

## ASPARAGUS WITH SLIVERED ALMONDS

*Asparagus is a lovely spring vegetable and so easy to prepare. It needs very little by way of flavor enhancement. The butter is great, but it isn't required.*

> 1 pound asparagus
>
> 1 tablespoon unsalted butter (optional)
>
> 4 tablespoons blanched slivered almonds

1.  Rinse the asparagus, then snap off the bottom few inches (wherever the spear breaks) and discard the tough bottom ends. Place the asparagus in a large skillet in a single layer and add ½ inch of water. Bring the water to a boil, then lower the heat to maintain a simmer and steam, covered, for 3 to 4 minutes.

2.  Drain the asparagus, add the butter, and toss. Serve immediately, with 1 tablespoon of almonds sprinkled on each serving.

Makes 4 servings.

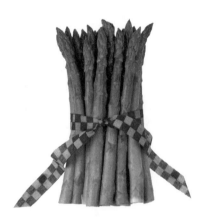

### Cleaning Leeks

Leeks, a member of the onion family, have a wonderfully sweet and delicate flavor. The only drawback is that they often have sand or dirt lodged between the layers. Here's an easy method for thoroughly cleaning leeks: Slice them in half lengthwise, then slice them crosswise. (In general, use as much of the green part as possible, discarding only the really tough, dehydrated, and ugly ends of the leaves.) Put the chopped leeks into a bowl of cold water and swish them around until they feel clean. Allow the water to settle for a moment, then fish out leeks with your hands and put them in a colander, leaving behind the sand and grit. After they've drained in the colander a bit, they're ready to be added to your dish.

# FRENCH TART WITH GREENS AND LEEKS

*This tart, inspired by a recipe in Patricia Wells's Bistro Cooking (1989), is excellent for using up leftover greens, broccoli, and the like. It makes wonderful picnic fare.*

Pastry Crust

    ½ cup brown rice flour

    ½ cup whole wheat pastry flour

    ½ teaspoon sea salt

    ¼ cup water

    ¼ cup extra-virgin olive oil

Leek Filling

    1½ pounds leeks (white and tender green parts), halved lengthwise, sliced, and cleaned (see page 160)

    ¼ cup water

    1 cup leftover cooked or stir-fried greens or broccoli

    3 extra large eggs

    ½ cup grated Parmesan cheese

1.  To prepare the crust, preheat the oven to 350°F and oil a 10-inch pie pan.

2.  Combine the flours and salt in a bowl and mix until well blended. Add the water and stir with a wooden spoon until the mixture resembles medium-size pebbles. Add the oil and stir until the dough begins to come together. Knead briefly in the bowl to obtain a moist dough. Press the dough out evenly in the prepared pan and smooth out the borders.

3.  Bake the crust for 10 to 12 minutes to dry it out somewhat, then remove from the oven. Leave the oven on.

4.  Meanwhile, prepare the filling. Combine the cleaned and chopped leeks and the water in a saucepan over medium heat, cover, and cook for about 4 minutes, until limp. Drain the leeks, transfer to a bowl, and add the leftover cooked greens. Mix well.

5.  Crack the eggs into a separate bowl and beat for about 30 seconds, then add the Parmesan cheese. Pour the egg mixture into the leeks and mix thoroughly.

6.  To finish the tart, pour the filling into the crust and bake for about 35 to 40 minutes, until the filling is firm.

    Makes 6 servings.

# COMPOSED SALAD WITH BEETS AND AVOCADO

*For a lovely meal, serve this with Rock Shrimp Potage (page 201) and corn on the cob.*

2 large beets

4 ounces mesclun or mixed baby greens

1 ripe Hass avocado

¼ cup Creamy Lemon-Ginger Dressing (page 229)

1. Leave the beets unpeeled; just trim away the greens and root, leaving 1 inch of stem and root. Put the beets in a saucepan, cover with water, and bring to a boil over high heat. Lower the heat and simmer, covered, for about 1 hour, until a sharp knife goes in easily.

2. Drain the beets, and once they're cool enough to handle, peel them with your hands under cold running water. Cut the beets in half top to bottom, then slice into thin half moons.

3. Divide the greens among 4 salad plates.

4. Cut the avocado in half lengthwise and remove and discard the pit. (An easy way to do this is to carefully drop a knife into the pit as if to cut it in half. Once the knife is stuck in the pit, twist gently and remove the pit on the knife. Attempt this only if you have a good knife and knife skills; otherwise just use a soup spoon.) Cut the avocado lengthwise into quarters and remove the peel. Cut each quarter into thin lengthwise slices and fan them around on the greens.

5. Arrange the slices from half a beet on each plate. Drizzle about 1 tablespoon of Creamy Lemon-Ginger Dressing over each salad and serve immediately.

Makes about 4 servings.

# RECIPES FEATURING PROTEIN FOODS

Try to eat two to three servings of protein foods daily to benefit the collagen matrix of your bones. The best choices are wild ocean fish, organically raised poultry or meat, and organic eggs; lentils, split peas, kidney beans, navy beans, black beans, and other beans and legumes, which are a good source of cholesterol-free protein, as well as calcium; and sunflower seeds, pumpkin seeds, almonds, cashews, and walnuts, which are all also high in trace minerals and essential fatty acids.

## What You Can Do to Prevent Food Poisoning

When preparing animal foods, it's important to attend to careful hygiene. After all, these foods won't help your bones if they make you sick. Here are some important guidelines:

1. Wash your hands well before handling *any* food. Use sufficient soap and dry your hands with a clean towel or paper towels. Always wash your hands again immediately after handling raw meat, chicken, fish, or other animal products. Do this before you touch anything else.

2. To sanitize cutting boards, countertops, and other surfaces, use a solution of 1 teaspoon chlorine bleach (any brand) in 1 gallon of water to wipe surfaces clean. Don't rinse these surfaces or dry them with a towel; just allow them to air-dry. To clean wood cutting boards (which should never be immersed in water), saturate a sponge with white vinegar and wipe the cutting board clean. To remove food particles from a wooden board without using caustic chemicals that could get into the food, sprinkle the board with coarse salt or baking soda, then wipe it clean with a clean damp cloth or sponge. Plastic boards can also be washed in the dishwasher. *Always* sanitize plates or cutting boards immediately after using them for raw meat, seafood, or poultry—before you put any other food on them. Even safer is to cut these foods on wax or parchment paper (perhaps the paper it came in), which can then be discarded.

3. To sanitize utensils, wipe or immerse them in that same bleach solution, 1 teaspoon bleach per gallon of water, or immerse in hot water (170°F or hotter) for a minimum of 30 seconds. A good dishwasher will normally reach these temperatures.

4. Wipe up spills of raw meat, seafood, or poultry, or their juices immediately, and sanitize the surfaces they fell on.

# Fish, Poultry, and Meat

Make sure the fish and seafood you consume are wild, not farm raised. Farm-raised fish sometimes have either very bland or off flavors; they may also be fed antibiotics or dipped in them. If you have a fish market nearby, this is probably your best bet for fresh, high-quality seafood. In terms of meat, poultry, and eggs, try to stick with organic, free-range, and grass-fed options. Commercially raised animals are usually given numerous antibiotics in their feed. Fortunately, there are now many natural food supermarkets and other stores that carry naturally raised poultry and meat, so we have more good options than in recent decades. Local farms can also be a good source of these foods. You can even buy grass-fed beef these days, hopefully from a local farmer, but if not, at some markets or even over the Internet. Use all seafood, meat, and poultry within 1 day of purchase unless it's frozen, in which case it keeps about 3 months.

# POACHED RED SNAPPER FILLETS WITH PARSLEY SAUCE

*Purchase a whole red snapper (about 1½ pound) or other similar fish, and have it filleted. Ask to have the head, bones, and tails placed in a separate bag so you can take them home to use for stock. To poach these delicate fillets, use fish stock from your freezer or make some using the snapper's bones and trimmings. These fillets should be served warm, so prepare the sauce first, then poach the fillets just before serving.*

> 2 cups fish stock (page 186)
>
> 1 teaspoon dried rosemary
>
> ½ teaspoon dried thyme
>
> 4 pods cardamom
>
> ¼ teaspoon sea salt
>
> 2 red snapper fillets
>
> 2 tablespoons Parsley Sauce (page 166)

1. Put the fish stock in a large, nonreactive skillet or poacher. Make a bouquet garni by placing the rosemary, thyme, and cardamom on a small piece of cotton cheesecloth and tying into a bundle. Hit it a few times with the handle of a knife or a big spoon to break up the spices slightly so they'll release more flavor. Add the bouquet garni and the salt to the stock, place the pan over medium-high heat, and cook until almost boiling.

2. Lower the heat to maintain a simmer and add the fillets skin side up. Poach gently, never allowing the poaching liquid to boil, for about 5 minutes. Turn the fillets over and continue poaching for another 3 to 4 minutes, depending on the thickness of the fillets. Test for doneness with a knife; if it goes through easily and the fish is white throughout, the fish is done. Gently lift the fillets out of the poaching liquid. (Discard the bouquet garni but keep the poaching liquid; you can add it to your fish stock stash.)

3. Top each serving with 1 tablespoon of the Parsley Sauce and serve right away.

Makes 2 servings.

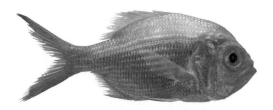

# PARSLEY SAUCE

*This lovely green sauce complements fish nicely, but is also wonderful on grain dishes, such as the Kasha with Mushrooms (page 208).*

2 tablespoons clarified butter (page 228) or unrefined coconut oil

3 tablespoons whole wheat pastry flour

1 cup hot fish stock (page 186) or vegetable stock (pages 181 and 182)

¼ teaspoon sea salt

2 tablespoons minced parsley

1 teaspoon freshly squeezed lemon juice

Freshly ground pepper

1. Heat the clarified butter in a small saucepan over medium heat, then add the flour, stirring continuously for about 3 to 5 minutes, until fragrant and lightly browned. Whisk in the hot stock, stirring vigorously with a whisk first, then with a wooden spoon, until the mixture thickens and is lump free. Bring to a boil, stirring all the while. Add the salt, turn down the heat as low as it will go, cover, and cook at a low simmer for about 10 minutes, stirring on occasion. If the sauce seems too thick, add a little stock or water.

2. Just before serving, remove the sauce from the heat and stir in the parsley and lemon juice. Season with pepper to taste before serving. Stored in an airtight container in the refrigerator, the sauce will keep for up to 2 days.

Makes about 1 cup.

# SALMON FRITTATA WITH FRESH DILL

*This is great for a light lunch or a hearty breakfast. For lunch, serve it with Oat-Dulse Crackers (page 211) or whole grain bread, and a mixed green salad. For breakfast, replace the salad with brine-cured pickles or sauerkraut (the kind with no vinegar). It's good cold, too. By the way, frittata is just a fancy Italian name for a thick omelet-like dish. If you want to finish the frittata under the broiler, use an ovenproof skillet.*

1 (7.5-ounce) can salmon (without oil or salt)

¼ to ½ teaspoon sea salt

2 teaspoons freshly squeezed lemon juice

1 tablespoon chopped fresh dill, or 1 teaspoon dried oregano or basil

Freshly ground pepper

2 eggs

1 teaspoon clarified butter (page 228), unsalted butter, or extra-virgin olive oil

1. Drain the juice out of the can and put the salmon in a bowl. With a fork, mash the salmon well to break up the flesh, skin, and bones. Add the salt, lemon juice, and dill and mix well, then season with pepper to taste.

2. Break the eggs into the salmon mixture and mix thoroughly.

3. Heat the butter in a skillet over medium heat, then pour in the egg mixture and smooth it out with a fork or a spatula. Turn down the heat to very low, cover, and cook for about 5 to 6 minutes, until set. The whole omelet should slide around if you shake the pan. Turn the omelet by sliding it out of the skillet onto the lid and then flipping it over into the pan. Cook for another 3 minutes. Alternatively, don't flip the omelet over; instead finish it under the broiler.

Makes 2 servings.

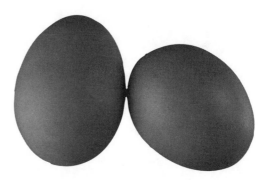

# SIMPLE ROASTED CHICKEN

*This makes for a delicious bone-healthy meal when served with Creamy Polenta (page 209) and Spiced Kale with Carrots and Turnip (page 149). Whenever you buy a chicken (always organic or free-range!), keep the backbone, neck, and wingtips for stock. Once you've cooked and used the chicken, save the bones for stock, too; you can freeze them if you won't be making the stock right away.*

1 organic chicken, cut up

1 tablespoon sea salt

1 teaspoon freshly ground pepper

1 teaspoon ground cumin

½ teaspoon ground ginger

1. Preheat the oven to 400°F. Line a large metal roasting pan with parchment paper.

2. Wash the chicken, pat it dry, and place it skin up in the prepared pan.

3. Put the salt, pepper, cumin, and ginger in a small bowl and combine thoroughly. Rub the mixture all over the chicken pieces, then pour about 1 cup of water into the pan. Bake for about 45 to 60 minutes, until the skin is crisp and the juices run clear when you poke a small knife into a thigh.

4. Serve the chicken hot. If you like, you can add a little hot chicken stock to the pan to pick up the browned bits and juices. Pour it back into your frozen stock stash, or use as thin gravy over the chicken.

Makes 4 servings.

## Uses for Leftover Cooked Fish or Chicken

- Add to any vegetable soup.

- Add to a salad.

- Make a sandwich with whole grain bread, salad greens, and a little salad dressing or good-quality mayonnaise.

- Add to stir-fried vegetables.

- Use as a quick snack with some celery and carrot sticks.

# PTCHA

*My husband, Bernie, finally got me his mother's recipe for ptcha (pronounced "pet-CHAH") so I could include it in this book. Ptcha is a savory gelled dish made from bones. If you serve it to European people born before 1940, you will probably thrill them. Others may not be so sure. Here's my version, which made Bernie very happy. Even though these types of gelled dishes have fallen out of culinary favor, they're extremely rich in bone-friendly nutrients, and their gentle texture finds favor with both children and the elderly. The gelling substances come from both bone and cartilage, which is why either chicken or calves feet, plus bones with some meat, are the preferred basic ingredient. A good concentrated beef stock—what the French call demi-glace—can also provide the gelling element. This version is quite garlicky.*

2 calves feet, coarsely chopped by the butcher, or 3 pounds meaty knuckle, knee, and shin bones

8 cups water

2 medium onions, quartered

½ cup white wine vinegar

1 teaspoon sea salt

1 bay leaf

Freshly ground pepper

6 cloves garlic

4 hard-boiled eggs

8 thin slices of lemon

Lettuce leaves

Sourdough bread

1. Combine the calves feet and water in a large saucepan over high heat, bring to a boil, uncovered, and boil for 10 minutes, skimming off any scum that floats to the surface.

2. Add the onions, vinegar, salt, and bay leaf, lower the heat, cover, and simmer for 4 to 5 hours, until the meat falls off the bone easily.

3. Strain the liquid into a clean glass or ceramic bowl. You should have about 4 cups. Remove the meat from the bones, chop it coarsely, and return it to the broth. (Discard the bones and other solids.) Season to taste with pepper and adjust the other seasonings as needed; it should be flavorful.

4. Mince the garlic, transfer it to a 9 by 13-inch glass baking dish, and gently pour the bone broth over the garlic. Chill in the refrigerator for about 20 minutes, until it begins to set.

5. Peel the eggs, cut them in half lengthwise, then gently press the halves into the *ptcha* in 2 straight lengthwise rows, distributing them evenly so that when the *ptcha* is cut into 8 servings, each will have an egg half. Chill for another 2 hours.

6. Serve cold as an appetizer on top of a lettuce leaf with a slice of lemon on top of each serving and the sourdough alongside. Pass the pepper grinder!

Makes 8 servings.

# PORTOBELLO BEEF STROGANOFF

*I love this recipe, especially served on top of cooked spelt pasta or hot polenta, with a salad on the side. You want to make it with grass-fed beef and full-fat yogurt, of course. Goat's milk yogurt is especially good here if you can find it. If you don't have a pressure cooker, don't worry; the stew can be cooked in a heavy, covered pot on the stove top over very low heat for about 1½ hours. Stir it once or twice and check to see whether you need to add a little more liquid.*

| | |
|---|---|
| 1 pound stew beef, in 1-inch cubes | ⅓ cup red or white wine |
| Sea salt | ¼ cup plain yogurt |
| Freshly ground pepper | 1 teaspoon prepared mustard |
| 3 tablespoons extra-virgin olive oil | 2 tablespoons unsalted butter |
| 1 large yellow onion, chopped | 6 ounces Portobello mushrooms, cut into ½-inch chunks |
| 1 small carrot, sliced | Cooked brown rice, whole wheat pasta, or polenta |
| 1 cup beef or vegetable stock, or water | |

1. Rinse the beef cubes and pat dry, then sprinkle them with salt and pepper. Heat 2 tablespoons of the oil in a pressure cooker over medium-high heat, add the beef cubes, and cook until browned. (Don't cover the pressure cooker at this point; that comes later.) If the beef releases some water, keep cooking until all of the water is evaporated and the cubes begin to stick and brown, about 15 to 20 minutes.

2. Heat the remaining 1 tablespoon of oil in a separate saucepan over medium-high heat, add the onion, and sauté for about 2 minutes, until translucent. Add the carrot and sauté for another 5 minutes. Add the stock or water, wine, yogurt, and mustard and mix well, then pour into the pressure cooker with the beef.

3. Place the pressure cooker over medium-high heat and stir the contents well to loosen all of the flavorful baked-on bits. Cover securely, bring up to pressure, then lower the heat, to maintain pressure and cook for about 25 minutes. Allow the pressure to come down naturally.

4. Meanwhile, heat the butter in a skillet over medium-high heat, add the mushrooms and ½ teaspoon of salt, and sauté about 6 to 8 minutes, until the mushrooms are wilted.

5. After the pressure is down, open the pot, stir, and then use a slotted spoon to remove all of the beef and some of the onions. Set them aside in a bowl. Pour the remaining contents into a blender and process until creamy. Taste and adjust the seasonings if need be, then pour the blended sauce back into the pot. Return the beef and onions to the pot, add the mushrooms, stir well, and reheat for 5 minutes. Serve piping hot over the rice, pasta, or polenta.

Makes 4 to 6 servings.

# Beans

Dried beans and peas are an excellent and often overlooked source of calcium, as well as superior sources of vegetarian protein and fiber. For optimum nutrition in vegetarian meals, combine beans with whole grains. Together, they provide complete protein, both soluble and insoluble fiber, magnesium, and all of the B vitamins except $B_{12}$. This combination is also an excellent source of complex carbohydrates.

Beans must be soaked, ideally for at least 8 hours, to eliminate phytates, compounds that can interfere with the absorption of minerals. Soaking also helps break down the abundant oligosaccharides in beans, the starchy molecules that cause gas. (If the ambient temperature is warm, it's best to do the soaking in the refrigerator.) Always discard the soaking water, then rinse the beans and cook them in fresh water to make them more digestible. If you forget or don't have time to soak the beans for at least 8 hours before use, you can streamline the process a bit. Combine the beans with a generous amount of water, bring to a boil, and simmer for 2 or 3 minutes. Then turn off the heat and let the beans sit, covered, for about 2 hours. Discard the water, rinse the beans, and proceed with the recipe. Certain spices, such as curry powder, cumin, and epazote, also help with the digestibility of beans, as does cooking the beans with kombu. In addition, it's important to chew beans thoroughly—at least 25 times per bite!—as the digestion of carbohydrates actually begins in the mouth.

For efficiency, consider making a big pot of plain cooked beans to use in soups, stews, salads, and other dishes. This will really cut down on the cooking time of recipes that call for them.

# ROOT STEW WITH WHITE BEANS AND WILD MUSHROOMS

*This great winter stew is delicious with Creamy Polenta (page 209). You might even want to double the recipe, as it keeps well in the refrigerator for several days. Should you get bored with it, add some extra stock and puree it all in the blender to make a creamy soup. You may be tempted to peel the burdock, but don't do it! The skin is highly nutritious, so just give it a good scrub. An alternative to julienning the burdock is to shave it by making numerous shallow downward cuts with a sharp knife all around. If you can't find burdock, replace it with ½ cup of julienned carrot; it won't be the same, but it will still be nice.*

½ cup white beans, rinsed and soaked at least 8 hours

2 bay leaves

¼ cup dried chanterelles or other dried wild mushroom

1 cup hot water

2 tablespoons extra-virgin olive oil

1 onion, diced

2 cloves garlic, minced

1 teaspoon dried thyme

1 teaspoon turmeric

2 carrots, diced large

1 (4-inch piece) daikon, diced large

1 small rutabaga, peeled, diced large

1 burdock root, julienned

1 cup vegetable stock (pages 181 and 182)

1 cup water

½ teaspoon sea salt

4 teaspoons chopped cilantro, for garnish

4 teaspoons chopped scallions, for garnish

1. Drain and rinse the beans, place them in a small saucepan, and add 1 bay leaf and enough water to cover by 1 inch. Bring to a boil over high heat, then lower the heat, cover, and simmer for 50 minutes, until tender but not falling apart.

2. Put the mushrooms in a small bowl, pour in the hot water, and let soak for at least 15 minutes.

3. Heat the oil in a soup pot over medium heat, then add the onion and garlic and sauté for about 2 minutes, until translucent. Stir in the thyme and turmeric, then add the carrots, daikon, rutabaga, and burdock and stir to combine.

4. Pour in the stock and water, then stir in the salt and the remaining bay leaf. Bring to a boil, then lower the heat, cover, and simmer for about 20 minutes.

5. Drain the mushrooms, reserving the soaking water, slice them thickly, and add to the soup pot. Add the mushroom soaking water, too, pouring it in slowly so that any grit remains behind in the bowl. Simmer 10 minutes longer.

6. Drain the beans and add them to the vegetables. Taste the broth and adjust the seasonings if you wish. Cover and simmer for another 15 minutes. Serve garnished with the cilantro and scallions.

Makes 8 to 10 servings.

# ANASAZI BEANS WITH COLLARDS AND SHIITAKE MUSHROOMS

*Anasazi beans are reputed to be good at lowering cholesterol. They are delicious plain, with nothing more than a sprinkling of chopped parsley or cilantro; they're also excellent in soups and dips. This dish pairs nicely with Rice and Millet Pilaf with Almonds and Cilantro (page 210) and Baked Buttercup Squash (page 155). Or be adventurous and try it for breakfast; after all, it's protein and calcium, just like milk.*

1 cup anasazi beans, rinsed and soaked at least 8 hours

1 bay leaf

1 tablespoon extra-virgin olive oil

3 cloves garlic, minced

4 large fresh shiitake mushrooms, stemmed and sliced

¼ teaspoon sea salt

Pinch of dried thyme

3 large collard leaves, stemmed and cut into 2-inch pieces

1 cup vegetable stock (pages 181 and 182)

1. Drain and rinse the beans, place them in a medium saucepan, and add the bay leaf and water to cover by 2 inches. Bring to a boil, then lower the heat, cover, and simmer for about 45 minutes, until soft. Alternatively, pressure-cook for 20 to 30 minutes and allow the pressure to come down naturally.

2. Heat the oil in a separate saucepan over medium heat, then add the garlic and sauté for 1 minute. Stir in the mushrooms, sprinkle salt and thyme over them, and sauté for about 4 or 5 more minutes. Stir in the greens and stock, then lower the heat and simmer, uncovered, for about 15 minutes.

3. Drain the beans, add to the greens, and cook about 5 minutes longer before serving. Alternatively, you can place the beans and the greens in two separate mounds on each plate.

Makes about 6 servings.

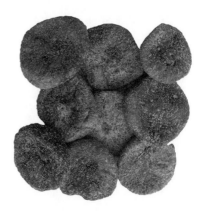

# MEDITERRANEAN HERBED CHICKPEAS

*Chickpeas are delicious and lend themselves to many dishes, both hot and cold. Because they take a very long time to cook, I always use a pressure cooker. If they are old and very dry, they may never get soft in a regular pot, but in my experience, a pressure cooker always does the job. Some people like to use canned chickpeas for convenience, but I prefer to cook them myself. This dish is great for a picnic or summer lunch and pairs especially nicely with fresh corn on the cob.*

> 1 cup chickpeas, picked over, rinsed, and soaked overnight
>
> 4 cups vegetable stock (pages 181 and 182) or water
>
> 1 (4-inch) piece of kombu
>
> ½ teaspoon sea salt
>
> 1 medium onion

Lemon Dressing

> 3 tablespoons freshly squeezed lemon juice
>
> 1½ tablespoons extra-virgin olive oil
>
> 1½ tablespoons flaxseed oil
>
> 1 teaspoon natural soy sauce (tamari or shoyu)

> 1 cup tightly packed parsley, minced

1. Drain and rinse the chickpeas, then put them in a pressure cooker along with the stock, kombu, and salt. Bring up to pressure, then lower the heat to maintain pressure and cook for 45 minutes, then turn off the heat and allow the pressure to come down naturally before removing the cover. Check that the chickpeas are soft; if not, continue cooking as long as needed.

2. Dice the onion and put it in a large serving bowl. With a mesh strainer or slotted spoon, remove the chickpeas from the water and add them to the onions while they're still hot. The kombu should be quite tender and may disintegrate; if not, chop it finely. Add the kombu to the chickpeas.

3. To prepare the dressing, combine the lemon juice, olive oil, flaxseed oil, and soy sauce in a small bowl or jar, and whisk or shake until thoroughly combined. Pour the dressing over the chickpeas while they're warm, and stir until well mixed.

4. Allow to cool to room temperature, then stir in the parsley. Serve immediately, or store in the refrigerator until ready to serve.

   Makes 4 to 6 servings.

# Soy Foods

Certain soy products are fine protein foods for people who aren't allergic or sensitive to them. However, I don't recommend soy milk as a regular drink. Soybeans contain goitrogens, or thyroid-lowering factors, and as a result, consuming unfermented soy products (tofu or soy milk) too often may interfere with thyroid function. Because they also contain certain substances that are estrogenic, they can help lower the incidence of hot flashes and other menopausal symptoms. On the other hand, these estrogenic substances may interfere with your hormonal system and may be contraindicated for people with hormone-sensitive conditions. I also don't recommended such highly processed soy products as texturized vegetable protein (TVP) and other ersatz meat products.

If you choose to eat soy products, do so no more than once or twice weekly, and use them in traditional forms, such as tofu, unpasteurized miso, and tempeh. Tofu and tempeh can be served in stand-alone dishes such as the two below. Miso is a great seasoning agent, especially for soups. It makes an appearance in several of the recipes in this book.

If you include soy foods in your diet, you'd do well to follow the example of the Japanese and also include ocean fish, other seafood, and seaweeds in your diet. All are high in iodine and therefore nourish your thyroid and counterbalance the soy. Iodine is an essential nutrient, utilized not only by the thyroid but also by all of the cells in the body.

# TEMPEH IN COCONUT MILK CURRY

*A nice vegetable protein dish, this will keep well for 3 to 4 days. The fats in coconut milk are very healthy, so don't sell yourself short by using low-fat coconut milk. Plus, full-fat coconut milk really brings out the flavors of the seasonings. Serve over long-grain brown rice.*

| | |
|---|---|
| ¼ cup dried porcini mushrooms | 2 tablespoons extra-virgin olive oil |
| 1 cup hot water | 1 medium onion, chopped |
| ¼ teaspoon cardamom seeds | 3 large cloves garlic, minced |
| ¼ teaspoon cumin seeds | 8 ounces tempeh, cubed |
| ½ teaspoon ground ginger | 1 cup coconut milk |
| ½ teaspoon curry powder | ½ teaspoon sea salt, or to taste |
| ½ teaspoon turmeric | 2 scallions, thinly sliced on the diagonal, for garnish |

1. Put the mushrooms in a small bowl, pour in the hot water, and let soak for at least 15 minutes.

2. Grind the cardamom and cumin seeds together in a mortar or spice grinder, then combine with the ginger, curry powder, and turmeric and mix well.

3. Heat the oil in a large skillet over medium heat, then add the onion and garlic and sauté for 1 minute. Add the spice mixture and sauté another 2 minutes. Add the tempeh in a single layer and sauté 4 to 5 minutes more, turning the tempeh over once.

4. Drain the mushrooms, reserving the soaking water. Chop the mushrooms, add to the tempeh, and sauté for another minute.

5. Add the coconut milk and salt, then add the mushroom soaking water, pouring it in slowly so that any grit remains in the bowl. Lower the heat, cover, and simmer for 25 minutes, stirring once or twice. Serve hot, garnished with the scallions.

Makes 4 servings.

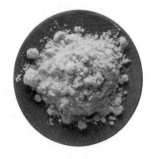

# COLD TOFU WITH GINGER AND SCALLIONS

*This is a terrific recipe when the weather is really hot and you need to cool off. While I generally recommend cooking tofu, in this case, as a hot weather antidote, it's fine to use it cold. Serve it as an appetizer, or with brown rice for a light lunch. Don't use silken tofu; the texture isn't right for this dish. Bonito flakes—dried flakes of aged pieces of a fish in the tuna family—are available in Asian markets and some natural food stores.*

12 ounces soft tofu

¼ cup natural soy sauce (tamari or shoyu)

4 teaspoons grated ginger

4 scallions, thinly sliced

4 teaspoons bonito flakes

1.  Fill a wide, 3-quart bowl with ice. Cube the tofu. I like to slice it into thirds horizontally, then into thirds lengthwise to end up with 9 batons, and then across into fourths. Put the tofu all over the ice in the bowl.

2.  Combine the soy sauce and ginger in a small bowl. Put the scallions in another small bowl.

3.  For each person, put 4 to 5 cubes of tofu in a small soup bowl, drizzle with ½ teaspoon of the gingered soy sauce, and sprinkle on the scallions and bonito flakes. Repeat as desired until all of the tofu is used up

Makes about 4 servings.

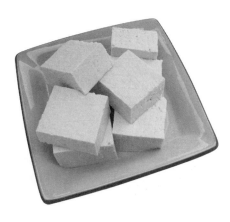

# COOKING WITH STOCK

Stocks can be used in cooking in a variety of ways beyond soups and stews. Try them in sauces and when cooking whole grain dishes. Basically, they can be used for the liquid in almost any savory dish. I've included recipes for a wide variety of fish, chicken, beef, and vegetarian stocks so you'll have a stock to complement any recipe. I've also included a section on soups and stews, below, to give you some ideas on how to put your mineral-rich stocks to use.

# Stock Recipes

Homemade stocks are an excellent source of minerals, as they are generally made with bones. While the muscles and organs of animals are very poor sources of calcium, bones are obviously an excellent source of bone-building minerals. They are not, however, easily edible. So how can we access their valuable nutrients? There are several ways.

The process of simmering stock will extract minerals from bones and seafood shells. You can enhance this extraction by adding a bit of vinegar or wine to the stock while it simmers. While many of us may not be eager to eat bones in their whole form, stocks made with bones and shells will enrich the nutrient value of any dish they're added to, while also deepening the flavor. Fine chefs devote a great deal of time and attention to their stocks. "My stocks are like gold to me," says Lauren Groveman, a cooking teacher in Westchester, New York, and author of *Lauren Groveman's Kitchen* (personal communication).

In addition to bones from fish, poultry, and meat and shells from seafoods, vegetable scraps can also contribute a well-rounded complement of minerals to stocks. Basic stock vegetables include onions, carrots, celery, leek and scallion tops, turnips, and parsley stems. For use in stocks, vegetables can be a little old, wilted, or ugly, as long as they're not moldy. Celery leaves are a great addition, but only use them in stock if the celery is organic; in conventionally grown celery, the leaves pick up much of the pesticides or herbicides, therefore it's best to avoid them. For that matter, it's best that all stock ingredients be organic, as the long cooking time will concentrate the pesticide and herbicide residues in conventionally raised foods. If you can't get organic bones, at least try to get bones from kosher animals.

When making vegetable stocks, always add a stick of kombu, a sturdy seaweed that's rich in minerals. To enrich any stock with even more minerals, add 1 tablespoon of agar flakes for each 8 cups of stock and heat until the agar is dissolved. Each tablespoon of agar contains 6 mg calcium, 8 mg magnesium, 6 mg folate, and a bit of iron (Hands 1990).

In making stock, avoid cruciferous vegetables, such as broccoli, cabbage, cauliflower, and kale; they are too sulfuric and create an unpleasantly strong odor when cooked for a long time. Also avoid the top ½ inch of carrots—the greenish bit where the carrot meets the leaf stem. That part is bitter and can give the stock a terribly harsh flavor that cannot be disguised. Onion skins are fine in stock, but they can cause the stock to turn brown. And unless you want a green stock, it's best to steer clear of parsley leaves. Here are a couple of lists to help you keep in mind which vegetables are good for stock, and which should be avoided because they have strong or bitter flavors or because they're deeply colored:

| Good Stock Vegetables | Vegetables to Avoid for Stock |
|---|---|
| Carrots | Beets and beet greens |
| Celery and celery tops (if organic) | Bell peppers |
| Garlic | Broccoli and broccoli leaves |
| Kombu | Brussels sprouts |
| Leek tops | Cabbage |
| Mushrooms (including the stems) | Cauliflower and cauliflower leaves |
| Onions and onion skins (which make stock brown) | Chile peppers |
| | Collard greens |
| Parsley stems | Eggplant |
| Scallion tops | Kale |
| Shallots | Kohlrabi |
| String beans | Mustard greens |
| Turnips | Parsley leaves |
| Zucchini | Potatoes and potato skins |
| | Sweet potatoes |
| | Yams |

For convenience, make big batches of stock—always at least 2 quarts—then freeze portions in different-sized plastic containers. Freeze some in ice-cube trays, some in pint containers, and some in quart containers. Once frozen, stock ice cubes can be placed in zippered plastic bags or other containers, to be retrieved as needed. Frozen stock keeps well for about 3 months. Vegetable, meat, or chicken stock can be kept in the refrigerator for about a week, but they must be brought to a boil every 3 days to eliminate any bacterial contamination. Fish stock should be frozen after 2 days in the refrigerator. Any time you thaw frozen stock it should be brought to a rolling boil; this will bring it to life, in a way, after its hibernation.

When making stock with bones, always add 1 tablespoon of vinegar or ½ cup of wine for every 2 quarts of water to help leach the calcium and other minerals out of the bones. (This need not be done with vegetable stocks.) The stocks I had analyzed ranged between 5 and 15 mg of calcium and between 3 and 9 mg of magnesium per 100 grams. On the whole, stocks are not a significant source of fats and contain no protein.

If you're new to making stocks, follow the recipes closely the first few times. As you become familiar with the process, don't feel bound by strict recipes, just follow the basic concept. Essentially, you start with a few vegetables and scraps, a bouquet garni (a bundle of spices and herbs), and, depending on the stock, some bones and vinegar or wine. Add enough water to cover by about 3 inches, and simmer with the lid ajar for several hours. Particularly with bone-based stocks, the longer you cook them the richer they get. You can leave the lid off for the last 30 minutes to concentrate the stock; that way it will take up less space in the freezer. Then you can dilute the stock a bit before using it in recipes. One important note: *Never salt a stock.* Because stocks are ingredients in other recipes, it's best that the salting be done in the final dish.

If you happen to be home for a day, you can make 2 or 3 quarts each of two different types of stock—say, vegetable and chicken—which can last you between a week and a month, depending on what you cook, how often you cook, and for how many people. I promise you that making stocks is worth the investment of your time and effort, in terms of both nutrition and flavor. Your health, and your bones, will be grateful.

## SIMPLE VEGETABLE STOCK

*This is an easy stock to make and have on hand. Sautéing the vegetables gives it a deeper and fuller flavor, but if you're in a rush you can skip that step.*

1 tablespoon extra-virgin olive oil

2 medium onions, chopped

4 carrots, top ½ inch discarded, chopped

3 stalks celery, chopped

1 leek, chopped and cleaned (see page 160)

10 cups water

1 (3-inch) piece of kombu

4 cloves garlic, peeled

parsley stems (no leaves) from 1 bunch parsley, about ½ cup

2 bay leaves

½ teaspoon dried thyme

1 teaspoon mixed white and black peppercorns

1. Heat the oil in a stockpot over medium heat, then add the onion, carrots, celery, and leek and sauté until the vegetables soften and become aromatic; don't allow them to brown. Add the water, kombu, garlic, parsley stems, bay leaves, thyme, and peppercorns. Bring to a simmer, then lower the heat to maintain a gentle simmer and cook for about 1 hour with the lid ajar.

2. Strain the stock through a fine-mesh sieve, pressing the solids with a wooden spoon to extract as much liquid as possible (but don't press so hard as to push the vegetables themselves through the strainer). Cool before storing in the refrigerator for up to 3 days, or in the freezer for up to 3 months.

Makes about 2 quarts.

# RICH VEGETABLE STOCK

*This stock will have a little oil in it from the walnuts and the olive oil, which are both rich in essential fatty acids. Don't try to remove it. This stock also has the unusual addition of beans. They must be soaked for at least 8 hours prior to making the stock, so plan ahead. Roasting the vegetables gives this stock a deep, rich flavor and a correspondingly deep color; however, you can omit this step if you prefer a lighter-colored stock.*

| | |
|---|---|
| 1 large onion, chopped | 4 quarts water |
| 2 carrots, top ½ inch discarded, chopped | 1 (5-inch) piece of kombu |
| 2 stalks celery, chopped | ¼ cup white beans, soaked for at least 8 hours |
| 1 medium leek, chopped and cleaned (see page 160) | ¼ cup parsley stems (no leaves) |
| 1 turnip, chopped | 1 bay leaf |
| 10 mushrooms with stems, sliced | 1 teaspoon dried sage |
| ¼ cup walnuts | 1 teaspoon dried thyme |
| 1½ tablespoons extra-virgin olive oil | ½ teaspoon peppercorns |

1.  Preheat the oven to 450°F.

2.  Place the onion, carrots, celery, leek, turnip, mushrooms, and walnuts in a large metal baking pan and drizzle with the oil. Toss well, until everything is evenly coated with the oil. Roast for about 20 minutes, until lightly browned, turning the vegetables every 5 to 6 minutes so they cook evenly.

3.  Transfer the vegetables to a stockpot and add the water and kombu. Drain and rinse the beans and add them to the stockpot as well. Add a little water to the baking pan to pick up the browned bits and juices, scraping the pan with a spatula or wooden spoon if needed. Pour this into the stockpot, too.

4.  Prepare a bouquet garni by placing the parsley stems, bay leaf, sage, thyme, and peppercorns on a piece of cheesecloth about 6 inches square and tying it into a bundle. Add the bouquet garni to the pot.

5.  Bring the stock to a boil over medium heat, then lower the heat to maintain a gentle simmer and cook for 1 hour with the lid ajar, skimming off any scum that rises to the surface. Remove the lid and cook 30 minutes longer to concentrate the stock.

6.  Discard the bouquet garni and strain the stock through a fine-mesh sieve, pressing the solids with a wooden spoon to extract as much liquid as possible (but don't press so hard as to push the vegetables themselves through the strainer). Cool before storing in the refrigerator for up to 3 days, or in the freezer for up to 3 months.

    Makes about 2 quarts.

# SIMPLE CHICKEN STOCK

*This stock is so easy. It requires very little prep and can be done in just half a day.*

   Carcass and bones of 1 cooked chicken, with or without skin

   1 medium onion, cut in half

   1 small carrot, top ½ inch discarded, chopped

   4 cloves garlic, peeled and smashed

   1 stalk celery, chopped

   12 cups water

   2 tablespoons brown rice vinegar or apple cider vinegar

   1 large bay leaf

   1 teaspoon dried basil

   ¼ teaspoon peppercorns

1. Combine all of the ingredients in a large stockpot over low heat, and allow to slowly come to a very low simmer. Continue cooking at a low simmer with the lid ajar for about 2 hours; don't allow the stock to boil. Remove the lid and cook for 1 hour more.

2. Strain the stock through a fine-mesh sieve without pressing on the solids; this will yield a very clear, unclouded stock. Chill the stock and then remove the congealed fat. Store in the refrigerator for up to 3 days, or in the freezer for up to 3 months.

   Makes about 2 quarts.

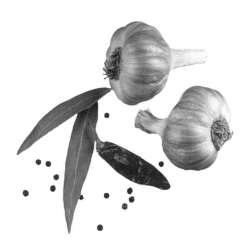

# GOURMET CHICKEN STOCK

*This delicious chicken stock has more ingredients and a richer flavor than the previous recipe. It takes a little more work, but it's worth it.*

2 bay leaves

½ teaspoon dried rosemary

1 teaspoon dried thyme

3 cardamom pods

1 teaspoon peppercorns

1 large onion, chopped

2 small carrots, chopped

2 stalks celery, chopped

1 small leek, chopped and cleaned (see page 160)

1 turnip, chopped

2 ounces mushrooms, sliced

2 tablespoons apple cider vinegar or balsamic vinegar

Back bones, neck, and wingtips of 1 chicken, washed, skin on

Carcass and bones from 1 cooked chicken

4 quarts water

1.  Prepare a bouquet garni by placing the bay leaves, rosemary, thyme, cardamom, and peppercorns on a piece of cheesecloth about 6 inches square and tying it into a bundle.

2.  Combine the bouquet garni and all of the remaining ingredients in a stockpot over low heat, and allow to slowly come to a very low simmer. Continue cooking at a low simmer with the lid ajar for about 5 to 6 hours; don't allow the stock to boil. Remove the lid and cook for 1 to 2 hours more.

3.  Discard the bouquet garni and strain the stock through a fine-mesh sieve without pressing on the solids; this will yield a clear, unclouded stock. Cool the stock overnight in a covered container in the refrigerator, then remove the fat from the top. Store in the refrigerator for up to 3 days, or in the freezer for up to 3 months.

Makes about 2 quarts.

# THE BEST AND EASIEST CHICKEN BONE STOCK

*Many thanks to Carol Kenney, one of the graduates of my Food Therapy Course, who passed this along to me. It's extremely easy to make, but you do need a 6-quart slow cooker. Here's the best part: The bones are surprisingly chewable and can be eaten straight, and you know you're getting a fabulous serving of natural organic minerals with each one. Whenever I make this stock, I eat one or two of the bones for breakfast every day for the following three days. Yum! Use the reserved meat to make chicken salad or a stir-fry with vegetables, or to make chicken soup. You can also make this stock with the bones from a roasted chicken. Just combine everything in the slow cooker and cook for 24 hours.*

> 3 pounds whole chicken legs with skin
>
> 2 bay leaves
>
> 1 tablespoon dried rosemary
>
> 1 teaspoon dried thyme
>
> 4 quarts boiling water
>
> ¼ cup organic apple cider vinegar, or ½ cup white wine

1. Combine the chicken, bay leaves, rosemary, thyme, and boiling water in a slow cooker, cover, and cook at the high setting for 4 hours.

2. With tongs, transfer the chicken to a large bowl. When it has cooled a bit, remove the meat from the bones and store it in a covered container in the refrigerator for another use. Return the bones to the slow cooker, along with all of the knuckle gristle and skin. Add the vinegar.

3. Cover the pot and cook on the low setting for 20 hours.

4. Strain the stock, reserving the bones and discarding the other solids. Store the bones in the refrigerator in a covered container. Cool the stock overnight in a covered container in the refrigerator, then remove the fat from the top and store in the refrigerator for up to 3 days, or in the freezer for up to 3 months.

Makes about 3 quarts of stock and 6 to 8 edible bones.

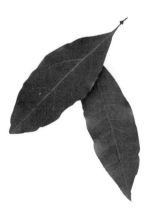

# FISH STOCK

*For convenience, you can purchase whole fish and have them filleted at the store. Ask to have the heads, bones, and tails placed in one bag, and the fillets in another. That way you can use the bones for stock and enjoy the fillets for several meals. Good choices of fish for this stock, known in France as court-bouillon, include snapper, bass, and sole.*

Heads, bones, and tails of two 10- to 12-inch mild fish

Greens of 1 leek

5 scallions, green parts only

1 large onion

1 carrot

¼ cup parsley stems (no leaves)

1 bay leaf

1 teaspoon dried oregano

1 teaspoon dried thyme

½ teaspoon peppercorns

4 quarts cold water

1 tablespoon apple cider vinegar or balsamic vinegar, or ½ cup white wine

1. Wash the bones in several changes of water until the water is no longer cloudy. Soak them in the last change of water while you prepare the vegetables.

2. Wash and chop the leek greens, scallion greens, onion, and carrot (discarding the top ½ inch of the carrot).

3. Make a bouquet garni by placing the parsley stems, bay leaf, oregano, thyme, and peppercorns on a piece of cheesecloth about 6 inches square and tying it into a bundle.

4. Combine all of the ingredients in a stockpot over medium heat. Bring to a boil, then lower heat to maintain a gentle simmer and cook for about 45 to 50 minutes with the lid ajar, removing the lid for the last 15 minutes of cooking to concentrate the stock.

5. Discard the bouquet garni and strain the stock through a fine-mesh sieve, pressing the solids with a wooden spoon to extract as much liquid as possible (but don't press so hard as to push any of the solids through the strainer). Use immediately, or store in the refrigerator for up to 2 days, or in the freezer for up to 3 months.

Makes about 2½ quarts.

# SHRIMP STOCK

*Obviously you would never discard the shrimp! It usually works the other way around. Several of the recipes in this book call for shrimp, or you may have other favorite methods for preparing them. In any case, anytime you have shrimp shells, store them in the freezer so you can make this delicious stock when you have the time.*

Shells and tails from 2 pounds medium shrimp (about 2 cups)

1 large onion, chopped

2 stalks celery, chopped

1 tablespoon peppercorns

⅛ teaspoon dried tarragon

1 bay leaf

2½ cups fish stock (page 186) or water

6½ cups water

½ cup white wine, or 1 tablespoon apple cider vinegar

1.  Wash the shrimp shells and tails, then combine all of the ingredients in a stockpot over medium heat. Bring to a boil, then lower the heat to maintain a gentle simmer and cook for 1½ hours with the lid ajar.

2.  Strain the stock through a fine-mesh sieve, pressing the solids with a wooden spoon to extract as much liquid as possible (but don't press so hard as to push any of the solids through the strainer). Use immediately, or store in the refrigerator for up to 2 days, or in the freezer for up to 3 months.

Makes about 2 quarts.

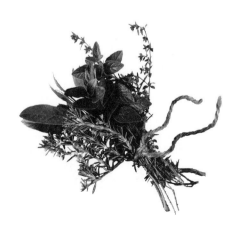

# BEEF STOCK

*Once you've made this stock, don't be so quick to discard the bones. The marrow that remains within is a rich source of calcium, fat, iron, and zinc. In fact, it has three times more calcium than milk, ounce for ounce. Although it's fallen out of favor as a food, marrow was an esteemed source of nutrients in the past. If you'd like to give it a try, blow or scrape it out of the bones after the stock is cooked, spread it on whole grain toast, and top with a little salt and white pepper.*

> 2 pounds beef marrow bones
>
> 4 quarts cold water
>
> 1 large carrot, top ½ inch discarded, chopped
>
> 1 medium onion, quartered
>
> 2 stalks celery, chopped
>
> 3 cloves garlic, peeled
>
> ½ cup parsley stems (no leaves)
>
> 2 tablespoons extra-virgin olive oil
>
> 1 cup red or white wine, or 2 tablespoons wine vinegar

1. Place the bones in a stockpot with the water, bring to a boil over high heat, and simmer for 10 minutes. Skim off as much of the scum as possible.

2. Add the carrot, onion, celery, garlic, parsley stems, oil, and wine, lower the heat to maintain a very low simmer and cook for 6 to 8 hours with the lid ajar, skimming occasionally.

3. Strain the stock through a fine-mesh sieve without pressing on the solids. Cool the stock before storing in the refrigerator overnight, then remove the fat from the top. It can be kept in the refrigerator for up to 3 days, or in the freezer for up to 3 months.

Makes about 3 quarts.

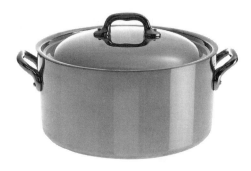

# RICH BEEF STOCK

*This is a great stock, but it takes some time and work. Make it on a chilly, rainy day; it will keep you warm!*

- 2½ pounds knuckle bones
- 6 quarts cold water
- ⅓ cup apple cider vinegar or white wine vinegar, or 1 cup white wine
- 2½ pounds beef marrow bones
- 2 pounds beef short ribs
- 1 cup water or white wine
- 2 medium onions, quartered
- 1 cup chopped carrots
- 1 cup celery tops
- ½ cup parsley stems (no leaves)
- 1 tablespoon crushed peppercorns
- 3 springs of thyme
- 2 bay leaves

1. Preheat the oven to 350°F. Place the knuckle bones and the 6 quarts of cold water in a large stockpot and allow to sit for about 1 hour. Add the vinegar.

2. Meanwhile, place the marrow bones and short ribs in a flameproof metal baking pan and roast for about 45 minutes.

3. Transfer the browned bones to the stockpot. Carefully pour off the fat from the baking pan, then put the pan on the stove top over medium heat, pour in the 1 cup of water or wine, and stir and cook for a few minutes to loosen up the browned bits from the pan. Pour this into the stockpot.

4. Bring to a rolling boil over high heat and skim off any scum that rises to the surface. After the scum stops rising to the surface, add the onions, carrot, celery tops, parsley stems, peppercorns, thyme, and bay leaves. Turn down the heat to medium-low and simmer with the lid ajar for 8 to 10 hours, skimming occasionally if needed.

5. Strain the stock through a fine-mesh sieve, pressing the solids with a wooden spoon to extract as much liquid as possible (but don't press so hard as to push any of the solids through the strainer). Store in the refrigerator for 1 day, after which the stock will be gelled. Use a thin spatula to carefully remove the fat congealed on top and discard. Store the stock in the refrigerator for up to 3 days, or in the freezer for up to 3 months.

Makes about 4 quarts.

# KOMBU STOCK

*Seaweeds are a wonderful source of minerals, but not everyone is fond of them. If you aren't a fan, this traditional Japanese stock is a perfect way to sneak some into your diet. Bonito flakes—dried flakes of aged pieces of a fish in the tuna family—are available in Japanese markets and some natural food stores.*

2½ cups water

1 (5-inch piece) piece of kombu

1 tablespoon bonito flakes

1.  Bring the water to a boil in a small saucepan, then add the kombu. Lower the heat, cover, and simmer for 5 minutes.

2.  Add the bonito flakes, turn off the heat, and let the flakes sink to the bottom of the pot. Let the stock sit a minute, then strain and use immediately. (The kombu and bonito flakes can be reused one time by simmering them in 2 cups of water for 10 minutes.) Use immediately in miso soup.

Makes about 2 cups.

# Soups

I love soups. When you're really hungry, there is nothing like a flavorful soup to soothe a growling stomach. In the heat of summer, chilled soups are cooling and refreshing, and in winter hot soups are comforting—and a time-honored defense against the common cold. Plus, soups can be an easy way to get people to eat their vegetables! Stock-based soups that contain no starchy ingredients such as flour, grains, or beans, are excellent alkalizers and can counteract the acidifying effects of breads, grains, and pastas. Therefore they are strong bone builders. If balanced by an alkalizing green salad, soups that contain starches or proteins, such as beans, fish, chicken, or meat (which are also acidifying), can also help the bones by providing a wide variety of nutrients. In addition, soups and stews are a great catch-all for odds and ends in the refrigerator. Sometimes the best soups are those made with various leftovers and some good stock—and they generally can't be duplicated!

Once you understand the basics of making soup, you'll come up with endless variations on your favorite recipes. Don't hesitate to experiment.

## CILANTRO EGG DROP SOUP

*Here is a quick, simple, and delicious soup. It makes for a nice light spring lunch when served with whole grain rye bread or crackers, Sardine Spread (page 225), and Asparagus with Slivered Almonds (page 160). Many variations are possible; just add ½ cup of any leftover cooked vegetable (chopped) or grain.*

2½ cups chicken stock (pages 183 and 184)

¼ teaspoon sea salt

1 egg, well beaten

2 tablespoons chopped cilantro

Freshly ground pepper

1. Combine the stock and salt in a medium saucepan over medium-high heat and bring to a boil.

2. Lower the heat to medium-low and slowly pour the beaten egg to the boiling stock, stirring continuously with a fork (to keep the egg in strands) until the egg is cooked firm and stands out from the stock, about 1 minute. Serve immediately, topping each serving with 1 tablespoon of cilantro and freshly ground pepper to taste.

Makes 2 servings.

# PINTO BEAN SOUP WITH DILL

*The beans must be soaked in advance, so plan ahead. The agar is optional. It won't add any flavor, but it will enhance the mineral content. For a more south-of-the-border flavor, substitute cilantro for the dill.*

1 tablespoon extra-virgin olive oil

1 medium onion, finely diced

1 small carrot, finely diced

2 stalks celery, finely diced

1 teaspoon ground cumin

1 teaspoon turmeric

4 cups vegetable stock (pages 181 and 182), chicken stock (pages 183 and 184), beef stock (pages 188 and 189), or water

1 tablespoon agar flakes (optional)

1 cup pinto beans, soaked for at least 8 hours

1 teaspoon sea salt

4 teaspoons chopped dill, for garnish

1.  Heat the oil in a soup pot over medium heat, then add the onion, carrot, and celery in that order, sautéing each for about 1 minute before adding the next. Add the cumin and turmeric, mix well, and sauté for another 30 to 40 seconds, then add the stock and the agar.

2.  Drain and rinse the beans, add them to the pot, and bring to a boil over high heat. Lower the heat, cover, and simmer for about 1 hour, stirring every 15 minutes or so. When the beans are soft, add the salt, and continue cooking for another 15 minutes.

3.  Serve hot, garnishing each serving with 1 teaspoon of the dill.

    Makes about 4 servings.

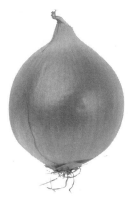

# GUMBO

*This is a meat-free variation on this popular Southern stew. If you want to more closely approximate the original dish, be sure to include the okra, and also add some cooked fish, seafood, or chicken at the end of the cooking time and then simmer for an extra 5 minutes. The buckwheat flour will give the gumbo a dark brown color and deeper flavor; use whole wheat pastry flour if you'd prefer a lighter dish. It's a great dish on its own, and also over rice or other grains, served with a salad or Basic Garlic Greens (page 147).*

2 leeks, halved lengthwise, sliced ¼ inch thick, and cleaned (see page 160)

1 cup onion, diced

1 small carrot, diced

1 stalk celery, diced

1 cup sliced okra (optional)

2 cloves garlic, coarsely chopped

2 cups vegetable stock (pages 181 and 182), fish stock (page 186), or chicken stock (pages 183 and 184)

1 bay leaf

¼ cup dried porcini mushrooms (optional)

3 tablespoons clarified butter (page 228) or unsalted butter

½ teaspoon cumin seeds

1 tablespoon filé powder

¼ cup buckwheat flour or whole wheat pastry flour

1 cup boiling water

1 teaspoon sea salt

Freshly ground pepper

1. Combine the leeks, onion, carrot, celery, okra, garlic, stock, and bay leaf in a soup pot over high heat. Break the mushrooms into small pieces and add them to the pot. Once the stock comes to a boil, lower the heat to maintain a simmer and cook with the lid ajar for about 15 minutes.

2. Heat the clarified butter in a small saucepan over medium-high heat, add the cumin seeds, and cook for a minute or two, stirring constantly, until fragrant. Add the filé powder and cook for another minute, stirring constantly, then add the buckwheat flour, and continue to stir and cook for 3 to 4 minutes. Slowly pour in the boiling water, whisking all the while, and continue to whisk until thick and lump free. Simmer for 1 minute, then scrape into the soup pot and stir well.

3. Stir in the salt, cover, and simmer for 10 to 15 minutes, stirring occasionally. Adjust the seasonings and serve piping hot, topped with freshly ground pepper.

Makes 3 to 4 servings, or more if you add cooked fish or chicken.

# AVOCADO-CUCUMBER SOUP

*This is a great cooling soup for a summer lunch, perhaps served with some steamed rock shrimp and corn on the cob. If you make extra, try something different and have the leftover soup for a refreshing breakfast on a hot day. The flaxseeds make this a good source of omega-3 and omega-6 fatty acids.*

1 clove garlic, peeled

1 small ripe Hass avocado

2 large cucumbers, peeled, halved lengthwise, seeded, and chopped

2 teaspoons freshly squeezed lemon juice, or 2 tablespoons umeboshi vinegar (see page 145)

4 cups chicken stock (pages 183-184) or vegetable stock (pages 181-182)

½ teaspoon chopped mint leaves, for garnish

2 tablespoons ground flaxseeds, for garnish

1. Remove the measuring cap from the lid of a blender, start the machine, then drop in the garlic and process until splattered against the blender wall.

2. Scoop the avocado flesh into the blender with a spoon, then add the cucumbers, lemon juice, and stock. Cover the blender and puree until smooth. Serve right away, garnished with the mint and flaxseeds. Serve cold for maximum cooling effect.

   Makes 4 to 5 servings.

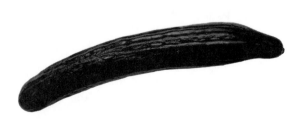

# COLD CUCUMBER-COCONUT SOUP WITH DILL

*Like Avocado-Cucumber Soup (page 194), this soup is wonderfully refreshing. If you have other uses for diluted coconut milk, you can mix an entire can of coconut milk with an equal amount of water. What's left over after making this soup can be stored in the refrigerator for about 10 days. It's a good substitute for milk or cream in cooking or even in tea or coffee.*

1 clove garlic, peeled

2 cucumbers, peeled, halved lengthwise, seeded, and chopped

½ cup coconut milk

½ cup water

2 cups chilled chicken stock (pages 183-184) or vegetable stock (pages 181-182)

1 tablespoon umeboshi vinegar (see page 145), or 1 teaspoon freshly squeezed lemon juice

¼ teaspoon sea salt

1 tablespoon chopped dill, for garnish

1 tablespoon shredded dried coconut, for garnish

1. Remove the measuring cap from the lid of a blender, start the machine, then drop in the garlic and process until splattered against the blender wall. Stop the blender.

2. Add the cucumbers, coconut milk, water, and 1 cup of the stock to the blender, cover, and process until well blended. With the machine running, remove the measuring cup again and slowly pour in the rest of the stock, along with the umeboshi vinegar and salt. Process for 5 minutes, until very creamy and smooth.

3. Adjust seasonings if need be, then pour the soup into a glass or ceramic bowl and refrigerate for several hours, until chilled. Serve garnished with the dill and coconut.

Makes 4 to 6 servings.

# CABBAGE AND CELERY SOUP

*Easy, warming, nutritious, and economical, this is the kind of soup I could live on. Serve it with Creamy Polenta (page 209; try the olive variation) and Mediterranean Herbed Chickpeas (page 174) for a nice light meal.*

> 1½ teaspoons extra-virgin olive oil
>
> 1 medium onion, chopped
>
> 2 cups shredded cabbage
>
> 1 teaspoon ground cumin
>
> 1 teaspoon sea salt
>
> 1 carrot, julienned
>
> 3 stalks celery, sliced thin
>
> 6 cups vegetable stock (pages 181 and 182)
>
> Freshly ground pepper

1. Heat the oil in a large saucepan over medium-high heat, then add the onion and sauté for about 2 minutes, until translucent. Add the cabbage, cumin, and salt, and sauté until the cabbage is wilted, about 2 to 3 minutes. Then add the carrot and celery and sauté 5 minutes more.

2. Add the stock and bring the soup to a boil. Then lower the heat, cover, and simmer for 35 to 40 minutes, until all of the vegetables are tender. Adjust the seasonings and serve piping hot, topped with freshly ground pepper.

Makes about 6 servings.

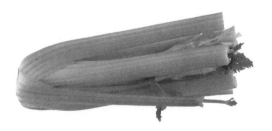

# MISO SOUP WITH WILD MUSHROOMS AND GARLIC

*If you like wild mushrooms, you'll love this simple, easy soup. Experiment with different types of dried mushrooms, or a combination. Shiitake, porcini, chanterelle, and maitake mushrooms are all good choices. For a truly special and very bone-healthy meal, serve it with Poached Red Snapper Fillets with Parsley Sauce (page 165), Yam Puree (page 156), Basic Garlic Greens (page 147), and brown rice. If this soup is too salty for you, add a little water at the end; if not salty enough, add some more miso.*

> 1 cup dried mushrooms
> 2 cups hot fish stock (page 186) or kombu stock (page 190)
> 4 cloves garlic, minced
> ¼ cup mellow barley or rice miso
> 1 scallion, thinly sliced on the diagonal, for garnish

1.  Put the mushrooms in a bowl, pour in the hot stock, and let soak for 45 minutes to 1 hour.

2.  Drain the mushrooms, reserving the soaking liquid. If using shiitakes, remove their stems (you can save them for stock). Slice the mushrooms into thin strips.

3.  Transfer the reserved soaking liquid into a 4-cup measuring cup, pouring it slowly so that any grit remains in the bowl. Add enough water to make 3 cups, then combine the liquid, mushrooms, and garlic in a large saucepan over high heat. Bring to a boil, then adjust the heat to medium-low and simmer, covered, for about 30 minutes.

4.  Combine the miso and ¼ cup of the soup broth in a small bowl and stir with a fork until smooth and creamy. Add the miso to the soup and simmer 2 minutes longer. Serve hot, garnished with the scallions.

Makes about 4 servings.

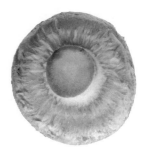

# CHICKEN SOUP

*This easy version of the universal comfort food is a rich source of alkalizing minerals.*

4 cups chicken stock (pages 183-184)

2 chicken thighs, without skins

2 carrots, peeled and diced

½ teaspoon sea salt

Freshly ground pepper

2 teaspoons chopped parsley, for garnish

2 teaspoons snipped chives, in ¼-inch pieces, for garnish

1.  Combine the stock, chicken thighs, and carrots in a medium saucepan over high heat and bring to a boil. Add the salt, lower the heat, cover, and simmer for 25 to 30 minutes.

2.  Remove the chicken thighs and, once cool enough to handle, take off the meat, pulling or cutting it into small pieces. Return the meat to the saucepan and freeze the bones for making stock.

3.  Continue simmering until the chicken is heated through, then adjust the seasoning if need be. Grind some pepper into each bowl, and garnish with the parsley and chives.

    Makes about 4 servings.

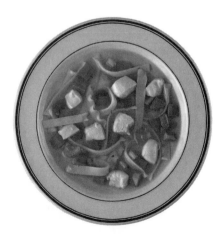

# SPANISH FISH SOUP

*This delicious and easy soup is excellent for company. Serve it over brown rice or kasha or with some good crusty whole grain bread, and accompanied by a side of Greek olives and a salad. Scrod is a good choice for the fish here, but any thick white-fleshed fish will do.*

2 tablespoons extra-virgin olive oil

1 medium onion, chopped

3 cloves garlic, chopped

¼ teaspoon dried tarragon

3 cups fish stock (page 186)

1 teaspoon sea salt

Pinch of saffron, crumbled

4 calamari (squid), cleaned and sliced into rings

½ pound small scallops

8 clams

1 pound fresh scrod

Freshly ground pepper

2 teaspoons chopped parsley, for garnish

1. Heat the oil in a large soup pot over medium-high heat, then add the onion, garlic, and tarragon and sauté for 2 to 3 minutes, until fragrant but not browned.

2. Add the stock, salt, and saffron and bring to a boil. Lower the heat, cover, and simmer for 20 to 25 minutes.

3. Add the calamari and simmer for 3 minutes, covered. Then add the scallops, clams, and scrod, and simmer another 5 to 6 minutes, until the clams have opened. Discard any clams that haven't opened within this time.

4. Ladle into bowls, then top each serving with pepper and a sprinkling of parsley.

   Makes about 4 servings.

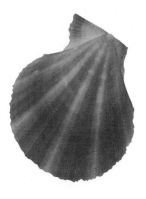

# HEARTY SHRIMP BISQUE

*This is a wonderfully luxurious soup, even without the cream usually associated with bisques. When you prepare the shrimp, save the shells for stock. Just throw them in a bag and store in the freezer for later use.*

3 tablespoons extra-virgin olive oil

½ cup minced onion

¼ cup finely diced carrot

¼ cup finely diced celery

¼ cup whole wheat pastry flour

½ cup white wine or water

3½ cups shrimp stock (page 187)

1 teaspoon sea salt

½ teaspoon dried thyme

1 bay leaf

24 shrimp, peeled and deveined

2 teaspoons snipped chives, in ½-inch pieces, for garnish

Freshly ground pepper

1.  Heat the oil in a soup pot over medium heat, then stir in the onion, carrot, and celery. Adjust the heat to low, cover, and cook for about 6 to 8 minutes, until the vegetables are soft but not brown.

2.  Increase the heat to medium, then sprinkle the flour over the vegetables, and stir until well combined. Continue cooking for 2 to 3 minutes, until the flour begins to give off a nutty aroma.

3.  Stir in the wine, stock, salt, thyme, and bay leaf, scraping up any flour stuck to the pot and stirring until everything is evenly incorporated. Bring to a boil, then lower the heat, cover, and simmer for about 15 minutes. Remove and discard the bay leaf.

4.  Add 20 of the shrimp and simmer for 2 to 3 minutes more, until they turn reddish pink. Puree the soup coarsely with an immersion blender, or in batches in a blender or food processor. Return the puree to the pot, simmer for another minute, then adjust the seasoning if need be.

5.  Prepare the remaining 4 shrimp for use as a garnish. Place them in a small saucepan with 1 inch of boiling water and cook until they turn reddish pink, about 2 to 3 minutes. Serve the soup hot, garnishing each bowl with a cooked shrimp and ½ teaspoon of chives. Pass the pepper mill!

    Makes 4 servings.

# ROCK SHRIMP POTAGE

*Rock shrimp is a warm-water shrimp from the Gulf of Mexico with a firm flesh similar to that of lobster and quite delicious. Because they have a very hard shell, they're sold shelled most of the time and therefore need no cleaning or deveining; plus, they cook very quickly. Although palm oil once had a bad reputation because of being so high in saturated fat, it turns out that the primary saturated fat it contains is palmitic acid, which seems to have a neutral effect on cholesterol levels. Unrefined red palm oil may be hard to come by, but it's worth looking for, as it has an incomparable flavor—and a great nutritional profile, being rich in beta-carotenes and other antioxidants.*

- 2 tablespoons red palm oil or extra-virgin olive oil
- 3 shallots, minced
- 3 cloves garlic, minced
- 1 tablespoon whole wheat pastry flour
- 2 cups hot shrimp stock (page 187)
- ½ teaspoon sea salt
- ½ pound rock shrimp
- ⅛ teaspoon freshly ground white pepper (optional)
- 1 scallion, green parts only, thinly sliced on the diagonal

1. Heat the oil in a saucepan over medium heat, then add the shallots and garlic and sauté for 2 to 3 minutes, until the shallots are translucent but not brown. Sprinkle in the flour and stir until well blended.

2. Stir in the stock and salt, then lower the heat and simmer for 10 minutes.

3. Add the shrimp and simmer for 2 to 3 minutes more, until they turn reddish pink. Serve right away, topped with the pepper and scallions.

Makes 2 servings.

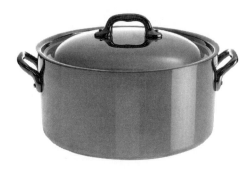

# SUNFLOWER SEED SOUP WITH CELERIAC

*And now for something completely different! Sunflower seeds are a rich source of calcium, magnesium, and especially zinc, all needed for healthy bones and hormone balance. Celeriac, also called celery root, is actually the root of a plant closely related to what we know as celery. Don't be scared off by its appearance; once you've sliced away that tough, knobby skin, what remains is crisp, white flesh with a pleasant flavor similar to a blend of celery and parsley. If you won't be using it right away, squeeze a bit of lemon juice over it or hold it in acidulated water to prevent browning.*

1 onion, diced

2 carrots, diced

1 celeriac, peeled and diced

1 small turnip, diced

4 cups vegetable stock (pages 181 and 182)

½ cup sunflower seeds

1 teaspoon sea salt

1 teaspoon umeboshi vinegar (see page 145)

1 tablespoon grated ginger

2 teaspoons chopped tarragon

1. Combine the onion, carrots, celeriac, turnip, stock, sunflower seeds, and salt in a soup pot over high heat. Bring to a boil, then lower the heat, cover, and simmer for 25 to 30 minutes, until all of the vegetables are soft.

2. Puree in batches in a blender or with an immersion blender until creamy. Then gently return to a simmer over low heat. Stir in the umeboshi vinegar, ginger, and tarragon, then taste and then adjust the seasoning if need be. Serve piping hot. This soup thickens as it stands, so dilute with stock or water as needed.

Makes 4 servings.

# QUICK AND EASY CONSOMMÉ WITH SOBA

*This is a great basic recipe for those times you need to put something together quickly.*

> 2½ cups beef stock (pages 188 or 189)
>
> 2 stalks celery, chopped
>
> ½ teaspoon sea salt
>
> ¼ cup broken-up soba noodles or other whole grain pasta
>
> ½ cup cooked beans or chopped cooked chicken or meat (optional)
>
> 1 scallion, thinly sliced, for garnish
>
> 2 tablespoons Basil and Cilantro Pesto (page 230; optional), for garnish

1. Combine the stock, celery, and salt in a small saucepan over high heat. Bring to a boil, then lower the heat, cover, and simmer for 5 minutes.

2. Add the soba and simmer 10 minutes longer.

3. Add the beans and simmer 3 minutes more. Serve hot, garnished with the scallions and pesto.

Makes 2 servings.

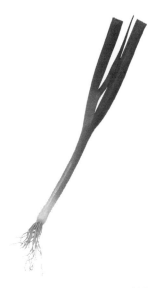

# WHOLE GRAIN RECIPES

Whole grains, such as brown rice, barley, oats, whole wheat, rye, and millet are the seeds of cereal grasses that have the germ, bran, and starch intact, as nature made them. When genuinely whole, as in not ground up, they can be planted or sprouted and new shoots will emerge, demonstrating their ability to create life. Refined grains, on the other hand, such as white rice, are missing both the bran and the germ and, as a result, most of their B vitamins, fiber, minerals, and vitamin E. And, obviously, they lack the life force that would allow them to sprout.

Because of their protective bran covering, whole grains are hard to digest, so they need good cooking in order to be soft and optimally digestible. For maximum digestibility, soak whole grains for about 8 hours prior to cooking. Use enough water to cover the grain by about 1 inch, and add about 1 teaspoon of something sour, such as lemon juice, apple cider vinegar, umeboshi vinegar, or even sauerkraut liquid or yogurt. (If the ambient temperature is warm, it's best to do the soaking in the refrigerator.) After soaking, discard the water and cook with fresh water. Soaking inactivates the phytates present in the bran, which can interfere with the absorption of minerals such as iron, calcium, magnesium, and zinc. Personally, sometimes I soak grains before cooking, and sometimes I don't; it's an optional step.

Remember that when consuming whole grains (as well as any other starches, including beans), it's best to chew each bite twenty to twenty-five times, since the digestion of starches begins in the mouth. Inadequate chewing can lead to gas, bloating, or abdominal discomfort a few hours after eating.

# FLAVORFUL RICE AND BARLEY

*This is a great basic cooking technique for whole grains such as brown rice, barley, millet, and quinoa. The grains should be soaked for at least 8 hours, so plan ahead. For a fluffier texture, add the stock boiling hot.*

½ cup brown rice

½ cup barley

2 cups water

1 tablespoon lemon juice or apple cider vinegar

2 cups vegetable stock (pages 181 and 182) or chicken stock (pages 183 and 184)

1 bay leaf

Pinch of dried oregano

½ teaspoon sea salt

1. Place the rice and barley in a bowl, add cold tap water, and swirl around well to loosen any dirt. Drain off the dirty water, catching the grain in a strainer. Repeat as necessary until the water runs clean.

2. Add the 2 cups of water and the lemon juice to the grains, cover, and soak for 8 hours or overnight.

3. Before cooking, drain the grains, then put them in a medium saucepan along with the stock, bay leaf, oregano, and salt. Bring to a boil over high heat, then turn down the heat, cover, and simmer for 1 hour.

Makes about 4 servings.

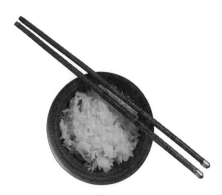

# CREAMY WHOLE GRAIN BREAKFAST PORRIDGE

*This excellent breakfast dish is savory, hearty, and satisfying; it's also very versatile. Try a mixture of two grains, such as barley and rice, or millet and quinoa. If you like, you can replace the sea salt and lemon juice with 2 teaspoons of umeboshi vinegar or natural sauerkraut juice. If you have leftovers, keep them in the fridge and reheat by steaming in a small pot with ¼ cup water per portion. Add a side of sauerkraut or cooked greens for some extra minerals. The grains are soaked overnight, so plan ahead.*

   1 cup whole grain, such as steel-cut oats or brown rice

   4 cups water, or 2 cups water and 2 cups mild vegetable stock (pages 181 and 182)

   1 teaspoon lemon juice or apple cider vinegar

   ½ teaspoon salt

   4 tablespoons almonds, chopped if you prefer

   4 tablespoons roasted sunflower seeds

   4 tablespoons flaxseed oil

   4 teaspoons maple syrup (optional)

1.  The previous evening, place the grain in a bowl, add cold tap water, and swirl around well to loosen any dirt. Drain off the dirty water, catching the grain in a strainer. Repeat as necessary until the water runs clean.

2.  Add 2 cups of the water and the lemon juice to the grains, cover, and soak overnight.

3.  In the morning, drain the grain, put it in a saucepan, and add the remaining 2 cups of water or stock and the salt. Bring to a boil over high heat, then lower the heat to maintain a very low simmer, cover, and cook for about 1 hour and 15 minutes without stirring.

4.  Top each serving with 1 tablespoon each of the almonds, sunflower seeds, and flaxseed oil, and 1 teaspoon of maple syrup if you wish. Stir well and enjoy!

    Makes about 4 servings.

# PLAIN KASHA

*This is easy and quick to make, and is a nice grain accompaniment to many dishes. Kasha, or toasted whole buckwheat, is a warming food, excellent for the cooler weather, and very popular in eastern Europe. It also seems to be less acid-forming than other grains, probably because it isn't technically a grain (the seed of a cereal grass), but rather the seed of a plant related to rhubarb. To reheat cooked kasha, steam it in ¼ inch of water or stock.*

> 2½ cups vegetable stock (pages 181 and 182) or chicken stock (pages 183 and 184)
>
> ¼ teaspoon sea salt
>
> 1 cup whole kasha

1. Combine the stock and salt in a small saucepan and bring to a boil.

2. Add the kasha, lower the heat, cover, and simmer for about 15 minutes, until all of the water is absorbed.

   Makes 5 to 6 servings.

# KASHA WITH MUSHROOMS

*This nice side dish is excellent winter fare. For a festive meal, try it topped with Parsley Sauce (see page 166) and served alongside Baked Buttercup Squash (page 155) and Simple Roasted Chicken (page 168).*

½ cup dried porcini mushrooms

2 cups warm water

Vegetable stock (pages 181 and 182), chicken stock (pages 183 and 184), or water, as needed

1 cup kasha

¼ cup sunflower seeds

½ teaspoon sea salt

1.  Put the mushrooms in a bowl, pour in the warm water, and soak for 30 minutes.

2.  Drain the mushrooms, reserving the soaking water, and chop them coarsely. Transfer the reserved soaking liquid to a 2-cup measuring cup, pouring it in slowly so that any grit remains in the bowl. Add enough vegetable stock to make 2 cups, then pour into a medium saucepan.

3.  Put the saucepan over high heat and bring to a boil. Stir in the mushrooms, kasha, sunflower seeds, and salt, then lower the heat, cover, and simmer for about 15 minutes, until the water is absorbed. Serve hot.

Makes about 4 servings.

# CREAMY POLENTA

*Polenta, made from coarsely ground cornmeal, is always a great side dish. I recommend organic polenta to avoid the varieties made with genetically modified corn. For a special treat, serve it with Root Stew with White Beans and Wild Mushrooms (page 172). Or, for a tasty variation, omit the salt, use olive oil rather than butter, and add ¹/₂ cup of pitted kalamata olives, stirring them in just before serving. Polenta is mushy at first, then stiffens as it cools. Here are several alternative serving suggestions: Pour the cooked polenta into a bowl, let it firm up for about 15 minutes, then invert it onto a plate and cut it into wedges. Or pour it into individual serving bowls or cups, then turn out onto individual plates after it firms up. You can even pour it into a loaf pan, refrigerate it overnight, then slice it and fry it for breakfast. You can also grill the slices after brushing them with a little olive oil.*

2½ cups vegetable stock (pages 181 and 182) or chicken stock (pages 183 and 184)

¼ teaspoon sea salt

½ cup yellow corn grits or coarse cornmeal

1 tablespoon butter or extra-virgin olive oil (optional)

1.  Combine the stock and salt in a saucepan and bring to a boil. Slowly pour in the corn grits, whisking all the while, then turn down the heat to low and stir continuously until thickened a bit, about 3 or 4 minutes. Cover and cook for 40 minutes, stirring often.

2.  Stir in the butter and serve hot.

    Makes about 2 servings.

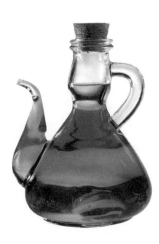

# RICE AND MILLET PILAF WITH ALMONDS AND CILANTRO

*This is a nice, flavorful side dish. It doesn't call for soaking the grain, but feel free to do so if you like. For a nice vegetarian meal, serve it with bean soup and a salad.*

½ cup long-grain brown rice

½ cup millet

1 teaspoon extra-virgin olive oil

1 teaspoon ground cumin

1 teaspoon turmeric

2¼ cups boiling chicken stock (pages 183 and 184) or vegetable stock (pages 181 and 182)

½ teaspoon sea salt

¼ cup coarsely chopped blanched almonds

2 tablespoons minced cilantro

2 scallions, thinly sliced

1.  Place the grains in a bowl, add cold tap water, and swirl around well to loosen any dirt. Drain off the dirty water, catching the grain in a strainer. Repeat as needed until the water runs clean.

2.  Heat the oil in a large saucepan over medium heat, then add the cumin and turmeric and stir and cook for 10 seconds. Add the grain and continue to stir and cook for about 4 to 5 minutes. Then stir in the boiling stock and salt, and bring to a boil. Lower the heat to maintain a very low simmer, cover, and cook for 45 to 50 minutes, until fluffy.

3.  Just before serving, add the almonds, cilantro, and scallions and toss to combine.

Makes about 6 servings.

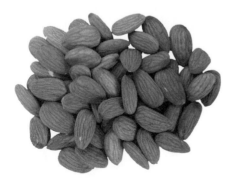

# OAT-DULSE CRACKERS

*These traditional Irish crackers are delicious with any hearty soup, and they keep well too. To make them more cookielike, add ¹⁄₂ teaspoon of baking powder to the flour mixture. Look for dulse, a type of seaweed, in natural food stores; the flakes are sold as a condiment. If you don't like the seaweed taste, use agar flakes instead. Agar is derived from a sea vegetable and is just as high in nutrients as dulse, but it has a very mild taste.*

2 cups oat flakes or rolled oats

1 cup sunflower seeds

½ cup whole wheat pastry flour

¼ cup dulse flakes

1 cup water

⅓ cup unsalted butter, melted

½ teaspoon sea salt

1 teaspoon caraway seeds or toasted sesame seeds (optional)

1. Preheat the oven to 350°F. Line a large metal baking pan with parchment paper.

2. Using a food processor, grind the oat flakes and sunflower seeds separately, until each has the texture of coarse meal. Pour both in a large bowl, add the pastry flour and dulse flakes, and mix well with a fork.

3. In a separate bowl, combine the water, butter, and salt. Whisk briefly to blend, then add to the oatmeal mixture. Stir well with a wooden spoon until everything is evenly moistened. The dough should have the texture of thick tuna salad.

4. Scoop out the oat mixture a tablespoonful at a time, placing each scoop on the prepared pan and pressing down with the back of a fork to make each cracker ½ inch thick and rounded. Sprinkle a few seeds over the top and press them in with the fork. Bake for 20 to 25 minutes, until browned around the edges, dry, and crisp. Cool before storing. Stored in an airtight container at room temperature, the crackers will keep for about 10 days.

Makes about 16 (3-inch) crackers. One serving is 2 crackers.

# PASTA WITH SARDINES

*Thanks to Susan Baldassano for the inspiration for this delicious recipe, based on the Sicilian classic pasta con le sarde. Sue, director of education and a cooking instructor at the Natural Gourmet Institute, specializes in Italian and other ethnic cuisines. The dish needs quite a bit of prep, so make it when you have some time to spare. It's totally worth it! Note that for bone health, you should never use skinless and boneless canned sardines. If other labeling doesn't clearly state this, check the nutrition label; the calcium content should be 20 to 30 percent of the RDA.*

Bread Crumb Topping
> 2 tablespoons pine nuts
> ½ cup whole wheat bread crumbs
> 4 anchovy fillets (packed in olive oil), minced
> 2 tablespoons extra-virgin olive oil

Sauce and Pasta
> 1 large beefsteak tomato
> Pinch of saffron
> 1 teaspoon fennel seeds
> 3 tablespoons extra-virgin olive oil
> 1 small yellow onion, finely diced
> 2 large cloves garlic, minced
> ½ bulb fennel, cored and finely diced
> 2 (3.75-ounce) cans sardines (packed in olive oil)
> 1½ cups shrimp stock (page 187), vegetable stock (pages 181 and 182), or fish stock (page 186)
> Sea salt
> 6 ounces whole wheat or spelt spaghetti

1. To prepare the topping, preheat the oven to 350°F (use a toaster oven if you have one).

2. Toast the pine nuts for 6 to 8 minutes, until lightly browned. Chop coarsely, then place in a medium bowl, along with the bread crumbs. Mince the anchovies, add them to the bread crumbs, then drizzle in the oil and stir until thoroughly combined. The mixture should be moist and resemble wet sand.

3. Transfer the mixture to a skillet over low heat and cook, stirring constantly, until toasty, fragrant, and slightly browned, about 8 to 10 minutes.

4.  To prepare the sauce and pasta, bring 4 quarts of water to a boil in a large pot. (First you'll use it to skin the tomato, but eventually it will be used to cook the pasta.) Make a few very shallow cuts through the skin of the tomato near the stem end and the bottom. Place the tomato in the boiling water for 30 seconds, then turn off the heat, remove the tomato with tongs, and transfer to a bowl to cool. When cool enough to handle, pull off the skin, cut the tomato in half crosswise, and squeeze out the seeds. Discard the seeds and skin and dice the tomato finely, discarding any unripe white pieces.

5.  Place 2 tablespoons of the hot water in a cup, crumble in the saffron, and set aside.

6.  Toast the fennel seeds in a small, dry cast-iron skillet over medium heat. Grind by hand in a mortar or spice grinder and set aside.

7.  Heat the oil in a saucepan over medium heat, then add the onions and garlic and sauté for 2 to 3 minutes, until the onions begin to soften. Add the fennel seeds and fennel, then turn down the heat to medium-low, cover, and cook until the fennel begins to soften and release its juices, about 10 minutes. Add the tomatoes, stock, and saffron, along with its soaking water, to the saucepan, raise the heat to medium-high, and bring to a boil.

8.  Remove the sardines from their cans, leaving the oil behind, put them in a bowl, and mash lightly with a fork. Add them to the sauce, stir well, then lower the heat, cover, and simmer for 20 minutes.

9.  Meanwhile, return the large pot of water to a boil, throw in about 2 teaspoons of salt, and then add the spaghetti and cook until al dente.

10. Taste the sauce, season with salt to taste, and simmer 5 minutes more. Drain the pasta, divide it onto individual plates, then top with the sauce and a sprinkling of the seasoned bread crumbs and serve right away.

    Makes about 4 servings.

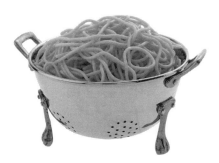

# RECIPES FEATURING FOODS RICH IN TRACE MINERALS

As mentioned in chapter 3, certain trace minerals are important for bone health: boron, manganese, zinc, copper, and silicon. While many foods contain various trace minerals, some are a good source of a broad range of these valuable nutrients, most notably seaweeds, nuts, and seeds. Vegetables and leafy greens, covered in the first section of recipes, are also excellent sources and make an appearance here in the form of green drinks.

All of the recipes in this section provide an abundance of trace minerals. Another approach is to add mineral-rich ingredients to other dishes. For example, you can add agar flakes to soups when you add the stock or other liquids, using 1 tablespoon per 8 cups of liquid. Another idea is to sprinkle seeds or chopped nuts on salads, grains, or practically any other dish.

# Seaweeds

Seaweeds are common foods throughout east Asia, as well as in northern Europe, Peru, the Philippines, and elsewhere. They are, however, unfamiliar at best to most North Americans, who are most likely to consume them in Japanese restaurants in miso soup, sushi, or nori rolls. In the natural foods world, these valuable foods are also popular, especially with those who follow a macrobiotic-type diet. Common varieties include kombu, nori, wakame, agar, and hijiki. Some people really don't like them, and others are quite fond of them. Give a few varieties a try and see what you think. They're very high in minerals, including calcium, iron, phosphorus, magnesium, boron, zinc, and over thirty others.

If you're hesitant to try seaweeds or not too fond of them, start by including them in stocks and condiments, as suggested in various recipes in other sections. But do try to be adventurous and eat them as featured ingredients, too, as in the recipes below, and in the Oat-Dulse Crackers (page 211). They're so rich that a little goes a long way, so it's not as though you'll be sitting down to a plate of seaweed! Your bones will thank you for your willingness to give it a try.

I do have one caution: If you use iodized commercial salt, consuming seaweeds could overload your body with iodine. One of the two should be avoided, and I suggest avoiding iodized salt and getting the mineral in a more natural form from seaweeds. I find it very interesting that in my classes people diagnosed with low thyroid function almost invariably love seaweed.

# CUCUMBER AND RADISH SALAD WITH WAKAME AND WALNUT-LIME DRESSING

*This cooling and refreshing salad is great summertime fare. Wakame, a seaweed that's a common ingredient in miso soup, is a wonderful flavor enhancer. It's very high in calcium and is also a good source of trace minerals and the antioxidant vitamins A and C. Look for wakame in natural food stores.*

1 ounce dried wakame

2 cucumbers (about 6 inches each)

6 large red radishes

2 tablespoons freshly squeezed lime juice

2 tablespoons walnut oil

1 tablespoon flaxseed oil

¼ teaspoon sea salt

1. Soak the wakame in about 3 cups of cold water for 20 minutes.

2. Peel the cucumbers, cut them in half lengthwise, and scrape out the seeds with a small spoon. Cut the cucumbers crosswise into ¼-inch slices and place them in a bowl.

3. Drain the wakame, cut away the tough middle rib, and chop the leaves very finely, then add to the cucumber.

4. Scrub the radishes well, cut them into quarters so the red shows, and add them to the bowl.

5. Whisk together the lime juice, walnut oil, flaxseed oil, and salt and pour the dressing over the vegetables, tossing thoroughly. Marinate for at least 1 hour before serving.

Makes 4 to 6 servings.

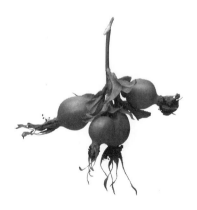

# HIJIKI CAVIAR WITH TOFU AND DRIED MUSHROOMS

*This is a powerful side dish; serve only 2 or 3 tablespoons per person. Try it as an accompaniment to Rice and Millet Pilaf with Almonds and Cilantro (page 210). It can also be served cold as a topping for a green salad.*

½ cup hijiki

¼ cup dried porcini mushrooms

¼ cup dried shiitake mushrooms

4 cups water

1 tablespoon light sesame oil

1 tablespoon minced garlic

1 tablespoon minced ginger

2 tablespoons natural soy sauce (shoyu or tamari)

8 ounces firm tofu, diced small

1. Soak the hijiki in about 2 cups of water for about 30 to 40 minutes. In a separate bowl, soak the porcinis and shiitakes in 2 cups of warm water for about 15 minutes.

2. Drain the hijiki, discarding the soaking water, and chop it very fine.

3. Drain the mushrooms, reserving the soaking liquid. Cut off and discard the stems, and chop the mushrooms coarsely.

4. Heat the oil in a skillet over medium-high heat, then add the garlic and ginger and sauté for 15 seconds. Add the chopped hijiki and sauté for 1 minute more. Add the mushrooms, soy sauce, and tofu, and then add the mushroom soaking water, pouring it in slowly so that any grit remains the bowl. Lower the heat and simmer, uncovered, for 15 to 20 minutes, until almost all of the liquid has evaporated.

Makes 6 servings.

# TOASTED NORI

*Cut toasted nori into strips and eat it straight, or rip it into small pieces and sprinkle it over cooked grains. Small children usually love this, and cats do too! Both can eat it easily because the nori is a blended composite of the sea vegetable, pressed together, so it disintegrates in the mouth.*

1 sheet nori seaweed

1. Toast the nori over a burner on the stove, holding it about 3 to 4 inches over the flame or heating element and moving it around until the entire sheet shrinks and turns dark, about 1 or 2 minutes. Alternatively, toast the nori in a toaster oven at the lowest setting.

## Mineral-Rich Garnishes and Condiments

You can always boost the mineral content of any dish or meal with the addition of mineral rich garnishes. These keep very well at room temperature for several weeks, so you can snack on them regularly.

## SHANA'S GRAIN-FREE NUTTY GRANOLA

*My daughter Shana came up with this idea, and I've adapted her recipe. My grandkids love it, and I love it too. These toasted nuts and seeds are rich in vitamin E and trace minerals and make for a delicious, if rich, breakfast or snack. A little bit goes a long way. Try sprinkling a handful on oatmeal or other hot cereals or using it as a topping for fruit salad. Even though the process isn't much work, it does take a long time, so plan to make it when you're home for the day. By the way, the soaking helps make the nuts and seeds more digestible.*

> 1 cup almonds
> ½ cup pecans
> ½ cup walnuts
> ½ cup sunflower seeds
> ½ cup pumpkin seeds
> 2 tablespoons maple syrup or agave nectar
> 1 tablespoon coconut oil, melted
> 1 tablespoon natural soy sauce (tamari or shoyu)

1. Place the nuts and seeds in a bowl, add enough water to cover by 1 inch, and soak for 7 to 8 hours or overnight.

2. Preheat the oven to 180°F and line a large baking pan with parchment paper.

3. Drain the nuts and seeds and spread them in a single layer in the prepared pan. Toast in the oven for about 2 to 2½ hours, stirring once or twice.

4. Combine the maple syrup, oil, and soy sauce and stir until well blended. Remove the nuts from the oven (leaving the oven on) and put them in a bowl. While they're still hot, pour in the maple syrup mixture and toss to coat well.

5. Transfer the nuts back to the baking pan, spread them out in a single layer, and return them to the oven. Continue toasting and drying the nuts for another 2 hours or so, stirring occasionally to break up any clumps and being careful that they don't burn.

6. Taste an almond. If it's reasonably crisp, turn off the oven and allow the nuts to cool; otherwise, continue cooking in 15-minute increments. Cool before storing in an airtight container. It will keep for several weeks, in or out of the refrigerator.

Makes about 3 cups.

# SESAME SEAWEED SPRINKLE

*This recipe requires the use of both a conventional mortar and pestle, and a suribachi, a Japanese mortar with ridges all around the bowl, making it ideal for grinding seeds. It's worth obtaining one (look in Asian markets and natural food stores), as a blender won't yield the same flavorful results. Use this as a condiment, sprinkled liberally over cooked grain dishes and vegetables. You can even eat 1 to 2 teaspoons per day straight, as a snack, pick-me-up, or mineral supplement. Wakame, perhaps familiar to you from miso soup, is one of the tastiest and most tender sea vegetables.*

½ ounce dried wakame

1 cup unhulled sesame seeds

1. Preheat the oven to 350°F.

2. Place the wakame on a baking sheet and toast in the oven for about 10 minutes, until dry and brittle. Remove from the oven and, once cool, break it gently into a mortar. Grind it with the pestle until powdery and discard any unbroken tough stems.

3. Wash the sesame seeds and drain thoroughly. Toast in a 1-quart stainless steel saucepan over medium-high heat, stirring constantly, until the seeds begin to pop energetically and become aromatic. Don't wait for the seeds to change color, as by then they might burn. (Don't use a skillet, as the seeds pop when they get hot and jump out of the skillet.)

4. Place the sesame seeds in a *suribachi* and grind for 2 to 3 minutes. Add the wakame powder and continue grinding for another 3 to 4 minutes, until 70 to 80 percent of the seeds are broken up. Stored in an airtight container it will keep for several weeks.

Makes about 1½ cups.

## Green Drinks

Sometimes it's hard to consume enough vegetables. Perhaps you don't have the time or inclination to cook them, or perhaps you're eating out a lot and the restaurants don't have enough appealing vegetable options. The following two recipes can give you a green boost and are easy to make as well as consume. Plus, they're packed with trace minerals. If you're worried about your bones and feel you don't eat enough vegetables, try them this way. And don't worry: You don't need an expensive juicer or other fancy equipment to make these green drinks. A countertop blender will work just fine.

### GREEN DRINK I

*This is my version of the calcium-rich vegetable drink that Nina Merer, from chapter 9, used daily to strengthen her bones. Ideally, all of the produce should be organically grown, for higher nutrient value and for better taste. Many variations are possible. Try adding half an apple, a couple slices of ginger, or a clove of garlic.*

> 1 carrot, chopped
>
> 1 small head romaine lettuce, bottom cut off
>
> 2 large bunches of parsley, washed and coarse stems removed
>
> 1 stalk celery, chopped
>
> 6 cups water
>
> 1 cup freshly squeezed orange juice (optional)
>
> 8 teaspoons flaxseed oil

1. Process the carrot, lettuce, parsley, and celery in batches in the blender, filling it just under half full and adding about 1½ cups of water each time. Process each batch until smooth, then combine all of the batches in a large bowl and mix well. Stir in the orange juice.

2. Just before serving, add 1 teaspoon of the flaxseed oil to each portion. Drink 1 or 2 cups each day. Stored in an airtight container in the refrigerator, it will keep for 3 days.

Makes about 8 cups.

# GREEN DRINK II

*This simple green drink is quick and easy to prepare in a blender, and a great way to start the day. Rudolph Ballentine, MD, author of Radical Healing (Ballentine and Funk 2000), says that cilantro is a natural chelator, which means it removes toxic minerals from the body. He recommends consuming about ¹/₂ cup per day. As with the other green drink, many variations are possible. Try adding some avocado, celery, arugula, or other greens.*

1 clove garlic, peeled

2 cups washed salad greens

½ cup packed parsley or cilantro

1 tablespoon freshly squeezed lemon juice, or ¼ cup freshly squeezed orange juice

2 tablespoons extra-virgin olive oil

1½ cups water

1 tablespoon ground flaxseeds

1. Remove the measuring cap from the lid of a blender, start the machine, and then drop in the garlic and process until fully minced.

2. Add the remaining ingredients, cover the blender, and process for about 2 minutes, until well blended. Drink immediately. If you let it sit, it separates, but you can just stir to reblend.

Makes 1 serving.

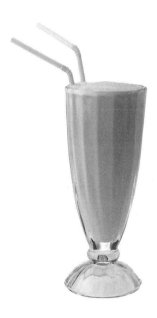

# RECIPES WITH EDIBLE BONES

Consuming edible bones is a time-honored practice for bone health. Did your mother or grandmother chew on chicken bones? Did your aunt use to love little fishes cooked crisp with their bones and all?

Canned salmon, often recommended as a source of calcium, only provides this mineral in abundance when the soft, well-cooked bones are consumed as well. So don't throw away the bones, eat them! When they include the bones, canned sardines are also a good source of calcium and other bone-building minerals. Fresh small fish with bones, such as sardines, smelts, and whitebait, are also a fine source of minerals, but with one disadvantage: For the bones to be edible these fish are usually deep-fried. While the high heat softens the bones and makes them edible, heating the cooking oil to such a high heat may damage it by oxidizing it, creating free radicals, which can contribute to cancer, atherosclerosis, other health problems, and aging in general, so it's best to eat fried small fish very sparingly. Fortunately, I've found a very satisfactory alternative method for preparing them: Just toss them with a little olive oil and bake them. Another good source of bone-building minerals is chicken wingtips and drumstick ends. If the chicken is roasted until well done, these parts are often so soft they can be munched on. In fact, some people really like to chew on all the bones for a while, which is an excellent idea—and good for the teeth, too.

You can also benefit from some of the minerals in the bones without eating them directly. Making stocks, explored in depth in an earlier section of recipes, is one way of extracting their minerals. Another way is to cook fish or chicken on the bone. During the cooking process, some of the bone minerals will migrate into the meat, so even if the bones aren't consumed at least small amounts of their nutrients will be available in the part you do eat. Other traditional mineral-rich dishes include gelled dishes made with bones or chicken feet (see the recipe for Ptcha, on page 169), and long-cooked stews in which the bones become soft and edible. And, fortunately for vegetarians, seaweeds are a wonderful source of minerals.

# FIVE-HOUR WHOLE FISH STEW

*This stew is a variation on the classic Japanese carp soup koi koku, which is traditionally recommended as a tonic and blood strengthener for women who have given birth. Because of the long cooking time, the fish bones are completely softened and become edible and quite delicious. This stew is a superior source of natural calcium and other essential bone minerals. In fact, according to the laboratory testing I commissioned, 1 cup provides over 800 mg of calcium and 50 mg magnesium, as well as about 50 percent of the recommended daily intake of vitamin D. Buy only the very freshest fish for use in this recipe, and ask that it just be cleaned, leaving on the scales, head, and tail, and cut it into 3 or 4 pieces.*

1 whole fish, such as pike, red snapper, or carp (about 1½ to 2 pounds)

4 thin slices of ginger

1 medium onion, diced

3 small carrots, diced or roll cut

1 cup white wine, or ¼ cup brown rice vinegar

6 cups water

¼ cup mellow barley miso

1. Rinse the fish well. Prepare the ginger by laying the slices on top of each other, then slicing them lengthwise into thin slivers.

2. Combine the fish, ginger, onion, carrots, wine, water, and miso in a pressure cooker over high heat. Bring up to pressure, then lower the heat to maintain pressure, and simmer very gently for 5 hours.

3. Allow the pressure to come down naturally, then open the pot and stir the stew vigorously to harmonize all of the flavors. Check the proportion of liquid, and if you'd like it more soupy, add some water. Find a bone and taste test; it should be easily chewed. If it's too hard, pressure cook for another hour. This stew can be kept in the refrigerator for 4 to 5 days. I don't recommend freezing it, because it kills the taste. Reboil each time before serving, adding a little stock or water if necessary.

Makes 6 to 8 servings.

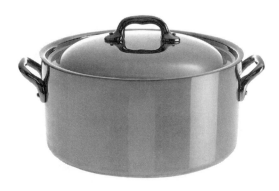

# CRISPY BAKED SMALL FISH

*This way of preparing small fish makes it easy to consume the bones. This version uses only ¹/₂ cup of oil instead of the 2 to 4 cups needed when they're deep-fried, as is traditional. I had this dish analyzed for mineral content, and a 3-ounce serving contained 117 mg magnesium, 327 mg sodium, 429 mg potassium, and a whopping 2,830 mg of calcium! This goes to show that eating bones is one of the best ways to get natural calcium. When you purchase the fish, have them cleaned, with the heads and tails left on.*

> 1 pound small whole fish, such as anchovies, smelts, or whitebait
> ½ cup cornmeal
> ½ teaspoon sea salt
> ½ teaspoon freshly ground pepper
> ½ cup olive oil or refined coconut oil
> Lime or lemon wedges

1. Preheat the oven to 400°F. Line a large metal baking pan with parchment paper. Wash the fish in several changes of water until the water runs clear. Pat dry with paper towels.

2. Place the cornmeal, salt, and pepper in a plastic or paper bag and shake until mixed. Add the fish to the bag and shake well until the fish are completely covered. Put the oil in a small, shallow dish and dip the fish in it briefly.

3. Put the fish in the prepared baking pan in a single layer and bake until they are crisp and dry but not overbrowned. Baking time depends on the size of the fish; whitebait takes only 20 minutes, whereas larger smelts may take 40 to 45 minutes. If the fish are longer than 3½ inches, turn them over once about halfway through the cooking process. Serve hot or warm as an entrée, appetizer, or snack, with 1 lime wedge per person.

Makes 3 to 4 servings.

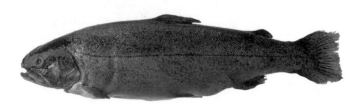

# SARDINE SPREAD

*This terrific spread for crackers can be used as an appetizer or as part of a light lunch. Tahini is a thick paste made from ground sesame seeds. You can find it in natural food stores and in the ethnic section of many supermarkets. Choose an unsalted variety. And, of course, the sardines should include the skin and bones; either packed in oil or packed in water is fine here.*

1 can (about 4.5 ounces) sardines

1 tablespoon grated onion

1 tablespoon freshly squeezed lemon juice

1 tablespoon tahini (optional)

1½ tablespoons chopped parsley

¼ teaspoon sea salt

4 rye crackers

Freshly ground pepper

1. Partially open the can of sardines, drain them, and then transfer to a bowl. Add the onion, lemon juice, tahini, parsley, and salt, and mash with a fork until well blended.

2. Serve atop the crackers, with a grinding of pepper on top.

Makes about 2 servings for lunch, or 8 when served on small crackers as an appetizer.

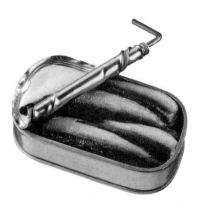

# WHITEBAIT FRITTERS

*After age ten, I grew up in a seaside resort in Argentina, where we ate all manner of fish and seafood, including fish livers. Tiny fish (whitebait), about 1 to 1½ inches in length, were very popular, always battered and fried. At the fishmonger in my New York City neighborhood, whitebait appear once or twice a year, and I always snap them up, a pound at a time. They are an excellent source of calcium and other minerals, as you eat the bones. Now my daughter Kaila lives in Christchurch, New Zealand, where whitebait fritters are a popular staple. This is an adaptation of a recipe from her boyfriend's mother, Linda O'Dea. If you want to make a bigger batch, increase all of the ingredients proportionately, but add only 1 extra egg for each additional 1/2 pound of whitebait.*

> 2 eggs
> 1 teaspoon whole wheat flour or spelt flour
> ¼ teaspoon sea salt
> Freshly ground pepper
> ½ pound fresh or frozen, thawed whitebait
> Butter for frying and for the bread
> Freshly squeezed lemon juice (optional)
> Whole grain bread

1. In a medium bowl, beat the eggs with a fork, then add the flour and salt and a few grinds of pepper. Mix to combine, then add the whitebait, and stir gently.

2. Heat a cast-iron skillet over medium-high heat, add a little butter, and swirl around to cover the base of the pan. Drop in spoonfuls of the whitebait and cook until the egg has set and the whitebait is turning white, about 4 to 5 minutes. Flip over with a spatula and cook on the other side for another 2 to 3 minutes. Season with lemon juice if you wish, and serve between slices of buttered bread.

Makes 2 servings.

# CRISPY BAKED CHICKEN WINGS

*Chicken wingtips are an excellent source of calcium and other good bone minerals. The trick is to chew on them really well and eat as much of them as possible, including the marrow. The wings need to be well roasted, almost dry, for the bones to get soft and tasty.*

1 teaspoon sea salt

1 teaspoon freshly ground pepper

2 pounds chicken wings with wingtips

Olive oil or refined coconut oil

1.  Preheat the oven to 400°F and line a large baking sheet with parchment paper. Mix the salt and pepper together.

2.  Wash the wings and pat dry, then rub them with the salt and pepper, place them on the prepared baking sheet, and brush with a little oil. Bake for about 50 minutes, until crisp, turning after 30 minutes.

    Makes 4 servings.

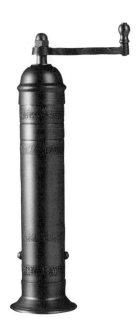

# RECIPES FEATURING HEALTHY FATS

Many of the recipes in this book contain some healthy fats, often in the form of olive oil or butter for sautéing. Here are a few recipes with more of a focus on healthy fats. Some are preparations you can use in other dishes, but there's also a wonderful pesto recipe and a couple of salad dressings. What could be healthier for the bones—and the entire body—than a big salad with fresh, seasonal leafy greens tossed with a dressing made with healthy fats, such as flaxseed and olive oils?

## CLARIFIED BUTTER

*A revered food in India, where it is known as ghee, clarified butter is also traditionally used in French cuisine as a standard cooking medium. Among its many advantages is that it doesn't go rancid easily and can be kept unrefrigerated in an opaque, airtight container for 2 or 3 months. (A stone pot with a tight-fitting lid works well.) It can also be kept in the fridge, but there it will become very hard. And because clarifying the butter removes the milk solids, it can be heated to a higher temperature than butter without smoking. For the same reason, people allergic or sensitive to milk protein can generally consume clarified butter.*

   1 pound unsalted butter

1.  In a small saucepan, heat the butter gently over low heat until melted, then continue simmering for about 10 minutes, spooning off the foam, which contains some of the milk solids. Remove from the heat and let stand for 3 minutes.

2.  Place a very fine-mesh sieve over a bowl or the container in which you'll store the ghee. Carefully strain the clear butterfat, leaving behind the water beneath the butterfat and the residue on the bottom of the pot. Store in an opaque, airtight container, and open only briefly when you need to access the contents.

   Here is another method. This one requires careful attention.

1.  In a small saucepan, cook the butter over low heat, simmering and letting it bubble until all of the water has been cooked out, about 20 to 30 minutes. Once that has happened, the butter will stop bubbling and the temperature will rise very quickly. The foam should be gone by this point. Remove from heat immediately, as the heat will rise and brown the milk solids. A little browning is nice, but too much is no good. Some of the milk solids may rise to the top.

2.  Strain through a fine-mesh sieve, leaving the milk solids behind.

   Makes about 1 cup.

## DR. CORSELLO'S SALAD OIL MIX

*Thanks to Serafina Corsello, MD, a pioneer of complementary and alternative medicine in the 1990s, for the idea for this salad oil blend, which is a great source of omega-3 fatty acids. Use this blend as the main oil in salad dressings. Because flaxseed oil is delicate and easily damaged by heat and light, keep the blend in an opaque bottle in the refrigerator.*

   1 cup extra-virgin olive oil
   1 cup flaxseed oil

I.   Mix the oils together in an opaque bottle and store in the refrigerator.

Makes about 2 cups.

## CREAMY LEMON-GINGER DRESSING

*The salad dressing is perfect for Composed Salad with Beets and Avocado (page 162). And it's so tasty that you won't have any trouble finding other uses for it. To make the ginger juice, grate about 1 inch of ginger root with a fine grater, then squeeze the juice out. A garlic press works really well for this; otherwise, just squeeze with your fingers. Don't use silken tofu here; it won't yield the correct texture.*

   4 ounces soft tofu, crumbled
   3 tablespoons extra-virgin olive oil
   3 tablespoons flaxseed oil
   3 tablespoons freshly squeezed lemon juice
   2 teaspoons ginger juice
   2 tablespoons water
   2 tablespoons chopped scallions, white parts only
   1 teaspoon sea salt

I.   Combine all of the ingredients in a blender and process until smooth and creamy.

Makes about 1 cup.

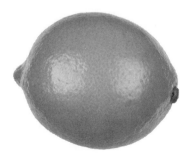

# BASIL AND CILANTRO PESTO

*Pesto is a great source of raw, highly nutritious greens, as well as good-quality omega-3 fatty acids. In addition to being a great pasta sauce, this pesto is also a terrific soup garnish. Soaking the walnuts makes them more digestible and enhances the availability of their nutrients; however, this step adds about 10 hours, so plan ahead. It's worth doing, as it helps get rid of that bite walnuts often have.*

½ cup walnuts

2 cloves garlic, peeled

4 cups loosely packed basil leaves, washed and spun dry

1 cup loosely packed cilantro leaves, washed and spun dry

1 cup extra-virgin olive oil

2 tablespoons white miso, or ¼ cup grated Pecorino Romano cheese

1. Soak the walnuts in 1½ cups water for 8 hours or overnight.

2. Preheat the oven to 200°F and line a baking sheet with parchment paper. Drain the walnuts, spread them in a single layer on the prepared baking sheet, then dry in the oven for about 2 hours. If they aren't dry at that time, return them to the oven for about 30 minutes more.

3. With the food processor running, drop the garlic into the work bowl through the feed tube. Stop the processor when all of the garlic is plastered against the sides, and remove the top.

4. Add the basil, cilantro, oil, and miso, replace the cover, and pulse the processor repeatedly until everything is well mixed, then run it for 1 minute or so to form a smooth, even paste. Scrape the pesto into an airtight container and store it in the refrigerator. The olive oil should rise to the surface and protect the pesto from contact with air, which can discolor the herbs. If need be, add a bit more oil to cover the pesto, which will keep for 2 weeks if covered by a layer of olive oil.

Makes about 2 cups.

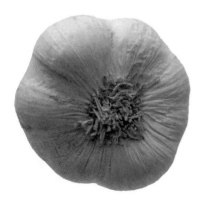

# DESSERT RECIPES

Surprise! Although desserts weren't included in my list of the seven top foods for bone health, I've provided a few recipes for them here because I know that for many people, dessert is the highlight of the meal. Unfortunately, or fortunately perhaps, I don't belong to that group, so whatever desserts I come up with are usually simple and don't take too long to make. On the whole, I don't believe desserts are truly food unless they're made with whole grain flours, fruit, and natural sweeteners. That said, a good dessert made with healthful ingredients can be really cheering and satisfying! In trying to come up with some genuinely bone-healthy desserts here, I looked for the most mineral-rich ingredients, as well as for ingredients high in essential fatty acids and fiber.

As tempting as traditional desserts may be, remember that white flour and refined sweeteners are acid-forming and can hurt your bones in the long run, whereas these recipes are more alkalizing and therefore support bone health. Speaking of sweeteners, I prefer maple syrup, malted rice syrup, malted barley syrup, fruit juices, and agave nectar. Let's take a quick look at these sweeteners, which appear to do the least damage to the bones:

- **Maple syrup**, which consists of sap from the maple tree boiled down and concentrated fortyfold, is quite rich in nutrients. In fact, 1 cup has as much calcium as 1 cup of milk. However, that doesn't give you license to drink a cup of maple syrup! Still, the abundant minerals buffer the acidifying effects of the simple sugars. It's also a great source of flavonoids, which have anticancer properties.

- **Malted rice syrup and malted barley syrup** are popular among whole foods enthusiasts. They're high in maltose, so they're good for people who want to avoid both sucrose and fructose. Both are mild and easy on the system.

- **Fruit juice and concentrated fruit juice** can be used as sweeteners, with the benefit of offering some extra nutrients. They contain many of the nutrients found in the fruit and are a good source of beneficial phytonutrients.

- **Agave nectar**, made from cactus, is one of the latest additions to the list of natural sweeteners. It has a low glycemic index, which means it provides sweetness without raising blood sugar levels too much. And it also contains inulin, a type of soluble fiber (Schepers 2007). It's sweeter than sugar, so you only need three-fourths the amount.

In truth, for a sweet taste after a meal, the simpler and more natural, the better. Beyond these recipes, healthful choices include dates, prunes, raisins, bananas, and natural applesauce with toasted almonds or sunflower seeds. Any fresh, seasonal fruit is, of course, an excellent choice.

# APPLE, STRAWBERRY, AND POMEGRANATE MOLD

*Feel free to try different juices and fruits in this recipe, with one caveat: Certain enzymes in raw (but not cooked) figs, mangoes, pineapple, peaches, guavas, papayas, and kiwis may prevent the agar from gelling, so they are not good choices for this dish.*

1¼ cups apple-strawberry juice

¼ cup pomegranate juice

½ cup water

¼ cup agar flakes

4 strawberries, sliced, for garnish

1. Combine the juices and water in a small saucepan, then sprinkle the agar flakes over the surface. Bring to a gentle boil over medium-high heat, then lower the heat and simmer for about 5 minutes, until the agar has dissolved. Beat with a whisk to ensure even dispersion.

2. Pour into a 2-cup mold and chill until set. To serve, unmold onto a plate and garnish with the strawberries.

   Makes 4 servings.

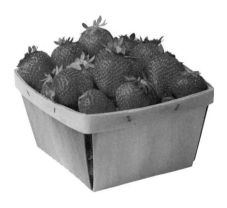

# ALMOND MILK PUDDING

*This is excellent either hot or cold. Kudzu, a starch extracted from the root of the kudzu plant, acts similarly to cornstarch or arrowroot but is preferable for bone health because it contains some calcium. It has a neutral flavor and creates a nice smooth texture when properly prepared. It's available in natural food stores, where you can also find apricot jam sweetened only with fruit juice concentrate, not sugar. And remember, it's especially important to choose organic citrus when you're using the zest.*

⅔ cup blanched almonds

2¼ cups plus 2 tablespoons water

1 teaspoon vanilla extract

⅓ cup kudzu powder

2 tablespoons maple syrup

Grated zest of ½ lemon

¼ cup fruit-sweetened apricot jam

Chopped toasted almonds, for garnish

1.  Grind the almonds in a coffee grinder, which makes them more fine and flourlike than a blender or processor would. Put the almond powder in a blender with 1½ cups of the water, and blend for 1 or 2 minutes, until smooth and milky.

2.  Pour the almond milk into a small saucepan over medium-high heat, bring almost to a boil, then lower the heat and simmer for 5 minutes. Strain through a fine-mesh sieve, put the almond pulp back in the blender, along with ½ cup of the almond milk, and blend and strain again. Return all of the almond milk to the saucepan, bring it back to a simmer, and stir in the vanilla.

3.  Combine the kudzu, ³⁄₄ cup of the water, and the maple syrup and lemon zest in a small bowl and stir until completely smooth. Add the kudzu mixture to the almond milk, stirring vigorously until thickened and lump free.

4.  Pour the pudding into 4 small ramekins. Mix the jam with the 2 tablespoons of water and spoon over the top of the pudding. Serve hot or cold, garnished with the chopped toasted almonds.

    Makes 4 servings.

# POACHED PEARS WITH COCONUT CREAM

*This is a lovely dessert for company. Thanks to Sally Fallon for the inspiration.*

3 cups water

1 cup sweet red wine, such as Madeira

2 tablespoons maple syrup or agave nectar

1 tablespoon vanilla extract

Freshly squeezed juice of 1 lemon

4 ripe Bartlett pears

1 cup Coconut Cream or Cashew Cream (recipes follow)

Toasted almonds or Shana's Grain-Free Nutty Granola (page 218), for garnish

1. Mix the water, wine, maple syrup, and vanilla in a saucepan over low heat; let it simmer while you prepare the pears

2. Put the lemon juice in a pie pan or large, flat-bottomed bowl.

3. One at a time, cut the pears in half lengthwise, core with a melon baller, cut out the stems, and peel the pear halves. Place them cut side down in the lemon juice and turn to coat with the juice to prevent browning.

4. Place the pears cut side up in a large, deep sauté pan over medium heat, pour the wine mixture over them, and bring to a low simmer. Lower the heat to maintain a gentle simmer and cook, covered, for 10 to 15 minutes, turning the pears over about halfway through the cooking time.

5. Allow the pears to cool in their cooking liquid. Serve them topped with Coconut Cream and garnished with a sprinkle of toasted almonds. If you'll be serving them the same day, you can keep them at room temperature until you're ready to serve. Stored covered in the refrigerator, along with their cooking liquid, the pears will keep well for 1 to 3 days.

Makes 8 servings.

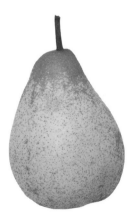

## COCONUT CREAM

*I found this great idea for a substitute for dairy whipped cream in cooking instructor Myra Kornfeld's book The Healthy Hedonist (Kornfeld and Hamanaka 2005). Here's my version, with one caveat: Don't use low-fat coconut milk; it won't yield the right texture.*

> 1 (14.5-ounce) can organic full-fat coconut milk
>
> 1 tablespoon agave nectar
>
> ½ teaspoon vanilla extract

1. Place the coconut milk in the freezer for 5 to 6 hours to allow the cream to rise to the top. Gently, without shaking the can, remove it from the freezer and carefully open it. Scoop the thicker coconut milk off the top and place it in a glass or stainless steel bowl. Scoop carefully; the thick part should go down about two-thirds of the way to the bottom of the can. Reserve the leftover coconut water for another use (you can always add it to a soup or stew).

2. Whip the coconut milk with a whisk or a hand mixer until thick, then stir in the agave nectar and vanilla. Stored in an airtight container in the refrigerator, it will keep well for several days.

Makes about 1 cup.

## CASHEW CREAM

*This is a fairly easy recipe, and one of my favorite dessert toppings. It has some protein, some calcium, and some fat, and is great to balance anything that has fruit or flour. Try it on the Fresh Fruit Salad with Toasted Sunflower Seeds (page 238) or the Whole Lemon and Coconut Custard (page 239).*

> 1 cup cashew pieces
>
> 1 tablespoon maple syrup or agave nectar
>
> ½ teaspoon vanilla extract
>
> ⅓ cup water

1. In a blender or food processor, grind the cashew pieces until pulverized, about 1 minute.

2. With the machine running, add the maple syrup, vanilla, and water and process until thick and creamy, stopping to and scrape down the sides if needed. If it's too thick, add another tablespoon or two of water. If too thin, let it sit for a couple of hours; it will thicken naturally. Use it all up the day you make it, as it doesn't keep well.

Makes about 1 cup.

# BROILED BANANAS

*This is one of my favorite quick and easy desserts, and everyone loves it!*

1 tablespoon clarified butter (page 228), unsalted butter, or coconut oil

2 bananas, cut in half lengthwise and once crosswise

2 tablespoons water

1 tablespoon maple syrup

1.  Preheat the broiler. Heat the butter in a cast-iron skillet over medium-high heat, then add the bananas and sauté on one side only for about 2 or 3 minutes, until soft and lightly browned.

2.  Mix the water and maple syrup together, then pour over the bananas. Place the skillet under the broiler for about 2 or 3 minutes, until the bananas begin to brown. Serve hot.

    Makes 2 servings.

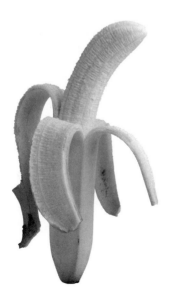

# MAPLE-WALNUT LOAF

*This low-carb treat is inspired by a recipe from one of the first natural foods cookbooks that I read, Beatrice Trum Hunter's Natural Foods Cookbook (1961). Because of the walnuts, it's an excellent source of omega-3 fatty acids.*

1½ cups walnuts

5 eggs, separated

¾ cup maple syrup

½ cup whole wheat bread crumbs or whole wheat matzoh meal

Grated zest of 1 lemon

Pinch of ground cloves

Pinch of ground mace

2 teaspoons vanilla extract

¼ cup fruit-sweetened strawberry jam (optional)

1. Preheat the oven to 325°F. Line a 9 ½-inch loaf pan with parchment paper, then lightly butter the paper.

2. Pulse the walnuts in a food processor until finely ground. In a large bowl, beat the egg yolks with the maple syrup for about 5 minutes, until thick and frothy. Add the walnuts, bread crumbs, zest, cloves, mace, and vanilla, and stir vigorously.

3. In a separate bowl, beat the egg whites with a whisk until they form almost firm peaks. For best results, use a copper egg beating bowl; you'll get much more volume. To determine if the whites are sufficiently stiff, lift the whisk and note how the egg whites stand up: If they bend over a lot, like a pointy cap bending down, they're not ready. If they bend over at the tip just about $1/8$ of an inch, they're ready. If they stand firm and straight up, they're overbeaten and run the risk of deflating really fast.

4. With a large rubber spatula, add one-third of the beaten whites to the bowl with the yolk mixture. Fold in by turning over very gently from the outside inward. Do not stir! Repeat twice more with the remaining whites. You should have a very light, fluffy batter. Pour it into the center of the prepared loaf pan and shake it very gently to distribute the batter. Bake the loaf without opening the oven for about 1 hour and 20 minutes. Test with a toothpick or thin knife inserted in the center: it should come out clean and dry. If not quite done, bake another 10 minutes.

5. Remove the loaf from the oven, run a knife along the sides, and invert the pan over a cake rack covered with parchment paper. Remove loaf pan and peel the parchment paper off the loaf. Cool. If desired, spread strawberry jam over the top of the loaf before slicing and serving. Stored in the refrigerator, the loaf will keep up to 1 week.

Makes 12 slices.

# FRESH FRUIT SALAD WITH TOASTED SUNFLOWER SEEDS

*This dish is so versatile: Serve it as an appetizer at brunch, for a summer breakfast, or as a light dessert. It's also a great way to use fruit that is beginning to get too soft. Any fruit you have available can be used, although I generally avoid using melons or watermelons because I find they make me burp. (Other people don't react that way, I know, so follow your own experience.) In the combination here, the juice oozing out of the orange wedges will help keep the apple from turning brown, and the banana lends a lovely soft, sweet flavor to contrast with the liveliness of the other fruits. Hopefully you're using organic apples, in which case you can leave the peel on.*

2 oranges, peeled and sectioned

2 apples, cored and cut in 8 wedges

1 banana, thinly sliced

1 cup seedless green grapes

1 cup raspberries or strawberries

1 cup blueberries

1 cup apple or orange juice

1 cup toasted sunflower seeds

¼ cup sherry (optional)

1. Cut the orange and apple sections crosswise twice, so that each wedge yields 3 pieces, and put them in a large serving bowl.

2. Add the remaining ingredients, toss, and serve. Alternatively, sprinkle the sunflower seeds atop each serving. Stored in an airtight container in the refrigerator, the salad will keep for 1 day.

Makes 6 to 8 servings.

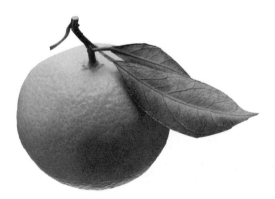

# WHOLE LEMON AND COCONUT CUSTARD

*This easy, low-carb dessert is very high in vitamin C and bioflavonoids, and a good source of essential fatty acids. Because it contains lemon zest, it has that delicious taste you get from good marmalade. (And because the peel is eaten, make sure you use an organic lemon.) This also makes a great pie filling. As I made it to my taste, it's not very sweet; add more maple sugar if you like it sweeter.*

> 1 whole Meyer lemon or thin-skinned organic lemon
> 4 eggs
> ½ cup maple sugar
> ¼ cup coconut milk
> ¼ cup water
> 1 teaspoon vanilla extract

1. Preheat the oven to 350°F. Grease the insides of 6 ramekins, or if you prefer, a 9-inch glass pie pan, preferably with coconut oil.

2. Scrub the lemon well, trim off the stem and tip ends, cut into wedges lengthwise, and once crosswise. Remove and discard the seeds and put the lemon pieces in a blender. Process briefly until broken up, about 30 seconds.

3. Add the eggs, maple sugar, coconut milk, water, and vanilla to the blender and process for about 1 minute, until homogeneous. Taste for sweetness and adjust if needed.

4. Pour the custard into the prepared ramekins or pie pan and bake for about 20 to 30 minutes, until lightly browned and firm in the center. Cool before serving. Stored in the refrigerator, the custard will keep for about 5 to 6 days.

Makes 6 to 8 servings.

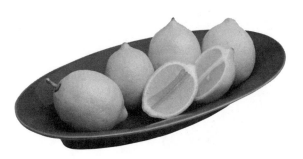

## FLAX-APPLE SHAKE

*Thanks to D. Marcus Johnson, who helped me test many of the recipes in this book, for this energizing recipe. Hopefully you're using an organic apple, in which case you can leave the peel on.*

¼ cup ground flaxseeds

1 apple, cored and chopped into a few pieces

½ banana, sliced

2 cups unfiltered apple cider or apple juice

1. Place the flaxseeds, apple, and banana in a blender, then add the apple cider. Blend first at low speed, then increase the speed to medium and continue blending until creamy.

2. Drink immediately.

   Makes 2 servings.

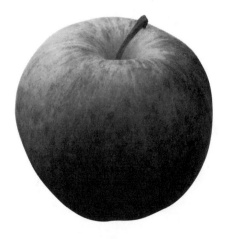

# REFERENCES

Abbott, L., J. Nadler, and R. K. Rude. 1994. Magnesium deficiency in alcoholism: Possible contribution to osteoporosis and cardiovascular disease in alcoholics. *Alcoholism, Clinical and Experimental Research* 18(5):1076-1082.

Abu-Id, M. H., P. H. Warnke, J. Gottschalk, I. Springer, J. Wiltfang, Y. Acil, P. A. Russo, and T. Kreusch. 2008. "Bis-phossy jaws": High and low risk factors for bisphosphonate-induced osteonecrosis of the jaw. *Journal of Cranio-maxillo-facial Surgery* 36(2):95-103.

Addington, S., N. Larson, and R. H. Scofield. 2006. Milk-alkali syndrome in pre-eclamptic pregnancy: Report of a patient and evaluation of albumin-corrected calcium in pre-eclamptic pregnancies. *Journal of the Oklahoma State Medical Association* 99(9):480-484.

Akhter, M. P., A. D. Lund, and C. G. Gairola. 2005. Bone biomechanical property deterioration due to tobacco smoke exposure. *Calcified Tissue International* 77(5):319-326.

Alhava, E. M., H. Olkkonen, P. Kauranen, and T. Kari. 1980. The effect of drinking water fluoridation on the fluoride content, strength and mineral density of human bone. *Acta Orthopaedica Scandinavica* 51(3):413-420.

American Society for Bone and Mineral Research. 2004. *ASBMR Bone Curriculum.* http://depts.washington.edu/bonebio/ASBMRed/structure.html. Accessed May 15, 2008.

Andrews, J. 2007. Surprise ingredients in fast food. NaturalNews.com, November 3. www.naturalnews.com/022194.html. Accessed April 5, 2008.

Appleton, N. 2005. Counting the many ways sugar harms your health. Mercola.com, May 4. http://articles.mercola.com/sites/articles/archive/2005/05/04/sugar-dangers-part-two.aspx. Accessed April 20, 2008.

Apsley, J. W. 2001. Biogenic medicine: Health care for the twentieth century. In *The Advanced Guide to Longevity Medicine*, ed. M. J. Ghen, pp. 45-56. Landrum, SC: Partners in Wellness.

Arnson, Y., H. Amital, and Y. Shoenfeld. 2007. Vitamin D and autoimmunity: New aetiological and therapeutic considerations. *Annals of the Rheumatic Diseases* 66(9):1137-1142.

Ballentine, R. 1978. *Diet and Nutrition: A Holistic Approach.* Honesdale, PA: The Himalayan International Institute.

Ballentine, R., and L. Funk. 2000. *Radical Healing: Integrating the World's Great Therapeutic Traditions to Create a New Transformative Medicine.* New York: Three Rivers Press.

Batmanghelidj, F. 1995. *Your Body's Many Cries for Water.* Falls Church, VA: Global Health Solutions.

Beall, D. P., and R. H. Scofield. 1995. Milk-alkali syndrome associated with calcium carbonate consumption: Report of 7 patients with parathyroid hormone levels and an estimate of prevalence among patients hospitalized with hypercalcemia. *Medicine (Baltimore)* 74(2):89-96.

Bellinghieri, G., D. Santoro, and V. Savica. 2007. Emerging drugs for hyperphosphatemia. *Expert Opinion on Emerging Drugs* 12(3):355-365.

Biglia, N., L. Mariani, L. Sgro, P. Mininanni, G. Moggio, and P. Sismondi. 2007. Increased incidence of lobular breast cancer in women treated with hormone replacement therapy: Implications for diagnosis, surgical and medical treatment. *Endocrine-Related Cancer* 14(3):549-567.

Bischoff-Ferrari, H. A., B. Dawson-Hughes, W. C. Willett, H. B. Staehelin, M. G. Bazemore, R. Y. Zee, and J. B. Wong. 2004. Effect of vitamin D on falls: A meta-analysis. *Journal of the American Medical Association* 291(16):1999-2006.

Black, D. 1988. *Health at the Crossroads: Exploring the Conflict Between Natural Healing and Conventional Medicine.* Springville, UT: Tapestry Press.

Blake, G. M., K. M. Knapp, and I. Fogelman. 2002. Absolute fracture risk varies with bone densitometry technique used: A theoretical and in vivo study of fracture cases. *Journal of Clinical Densitometry* 5(2):109-116.

Bolland, M. J., P. A. Barber, R. N. Doughty, B. Mason, A. Horne, R. Ames, G. D. Gamble, A. Grey, and I. R. Reid. 2008. Vascular events in healthy older women receiving calcium supplementation: Randomised controlled trial. *British Medical Journal* 336(7638):262-266.

Bonnick, S. L. 2006. Osteoporosis in men and women. *Clinical Cornerstone* 8(1):28-39.

Booth, S. L. 2007. Vitamin K status in the elderly. *Current Opinion in Clinical Nutrition and Metabolic Care* 10(1):20-23.

Booth, S. L., and J. Mayer. 2000. Warfarin use and fracture risk. *Nutrition Reviews* 58(1):20-22.

Boscoe, F. P., and M. J. Schymura. 2006. Solar ultraviolet-B exposure and cancer incidence and mortality in the United States, 1993-2002. *BioMed Central Cancer* 6:264.

Brody, J. 1997. Personal Health column. *New York Times*, September 30. http://query.nytimes.com/gst/fullpage.html?res=9806E3DC133AF933A0575AC0A961958260. Accessed April 5, 2008.

Bruinsma, K., and D. L. Taren. 1999. Chocolate: Food or drug? *Journal of the American Dietetic Association* 99(10):1249-1256.

Brunet, M. 2005. Female athlete triad. *Clinics in Sports Medicine* 24(3):623-36, ix.

Buckwalter, J. A., M. J. Glimcher, R. R. Cooper, and R. Recker. 1996. Bone biology. II: Formation, form, modeling, remodeling, and regulation of cell function. *Instructional Course Lectures* 45:387-399.

Campbell, T. C., and T. M. Campbell. 2005. *The China Study: The Most Comprehensive Study of Nutrition Ever Conducted and the Startling Implications for Diet, Weight Loss and Long-Term Health.* Dallas: Benbella Books.

Carmichael, K. A., M. D. Fallon, M. Dalinka, F. S. Kaplan, L. Axel, and J. G. Haddad. 1984. Osteomalacia and osteitis fibrosa in a man ingesting aluminum hydroxide antacid. *American Journal of Medicine* 76(6):1137-1143.

Caruso, D. B. 2004. Maker of Equal Sues Marketer of Splenda. Associated Press, December 1.

Cauley, J. A., F. L. Lucas, L. H. Kuller, M. T. Vogt, W. S. Browner, and S. R. Cummings. 1996. Bone mineral density and risk of breast cancer in older women: The study of osteoporotic fractures. *Journal of the American Medical Association* 276(17):1404-1408.

Chen, T. C., A. Shao, H. Heath III, and M. F. Holick. 1993. An update on the vitamin D content of fortified milk from the United States and Canada. *New England Journal of Medicine* 239(20):1507.

Childers, N. F. 1999. *Arthritis—Childers' Diet That Stops It! The Nightshades, Ill Health, Aging, and Shorter Life.* Gainesville, FL: Dr. Norman F. Childers Publications.

Childers, N. F. 2002. Apparent relation of nightshades (*Solanaceae*) to Arthritis and Other Health Problems. *Journal of Applied Nutrition* 52(1):2-10.

Cohen, A. J., and F. J. Roe. 2000. Review of risk factors for osteoporosis with particular reference to a possible aetiological role of dietary salt. *Food and Chemical Toxicology* 38(2-3):237-253.

Colbin, A. 1999. Osteoporosis: Preventing bone loss without drugs. *What Doctors Don't Tell You* 9(10):1-5. Available in part at www.wddty.com/03363800373023325932/preventing-bone-loss-without-drugs.html. Accessed May 1, 2008.

Cooper, C., E. J. Atkinson, H. W. Wahner, W. M. O'Fallon, B. L. Riggs, H. L. Judd, and L. J. Melton. 1992. Is caffeine consumption a risk factor for osteoporosis? *Journal of Bones and Mineral Research* 7(4):465-471.

Cotrozzi, G., and P. Relli. 1994. Osteoporosis. Current advances in etiopathogenesis, diagnosis and therapy: I. Etiopathogenesis and diagnosis. [In Italian.] *Clinica Terapeutica* 144(3):251-263.

Crayhon, R. 1994. *Robert Crayhon's Nutrition Made Simple: A Comprehensive Guide to the Latest Findings in Optimal Nutrition.* New York: M. Evans and Company.

Cumming, R. G., S. R. Cummings, M. C. Nevitt, J. Scott, K. E. Ensrud, T. M. Vogt, and K. Fox. 1997. Calcium intake and fracture risk: Results from the study of osteoporotic fractures. *American Journal of Epidemiology* 145(10):926-934.

Cummings, S. R., A. V. Schwartz, and D. M. Black. 2007. Alendronate and atrial fibrillation. *New England Journal of Medicine* 356(18):1895-1896.

Daniells, S. 2007. Are organic tomatoes more nutritious? Foodnavigator.com. July 5. www.foodnavigator.com/news/ng.asp?n=77947-organic-tomatoes-flavonoids. Accessed April 21, 2008.

Dawson-Hughes, B., S. S. Harris, H. Rasmussen, L. Song, and G. E. Dallal. 2004. Effect of dietary protein supplements on calcium excretion in healthy older men and women. *Journal of Clinical Endocrinology and Metabolism* 89(3):1169-1173.

Devine, A., R. A. Criddle, I. M. Dick, D. A. Kerr, and R. L. Prince. 1995. A longitudinal study of the effect of sodium and calcium intakes on regional bone density in postmenopausal women. *American Journal of Clinical Nutrition* 62(4):740-745.

De Vrese, M., A. Stegelmann, B. Richter, S. Fenselau, C. Laue, and J. Schrezenmeir. 2001. Probiotics: Compensation for lactase insufficiency. *American Journal of Clinical Nutrition* 73(2 suppl.):421S-429S.

De Vries, A. 1952. *Primitive Man and His Food.* Chicago: Chandler Book Company.

Di Costanzo, D. 1995. Fruit smoothie. *Self,* July, 133.

Elliott, R. B., D. P. Harris, J. P. Hill, N. J. Bibby, and H. E. Wasmuth. 1999. Type I (insulin-dependent) diabetes mellitus and cow milk: Casein variant consumption. *Diabetologia* 42(3):292-296.

Ellis, F. R., S. Holesh, and J. W. Ellis. 1972. Incidence of osteoporosis in vegetarians and omnivores. *American Journal of Clinical Nutrition* 25(6):555-558.

Enig, M. G. 2000. *Know Your Fats: The Complete Primer for Understanding the Nutrition of Fats, Oils, and Cholesterol.* Silver Spring, MD: Bethesda Press.

Enig, M. G., and S. Fallon. 2005. *Eat Fat, Lose Fat.* New York: Hudson Street Press.

Erasmus, U. 1993. *Fats That Heal, Fats That Kill: The Complete Guide to Fats, Oils, Cholesterol, and Human Health.* Burnaby, BC: Alive Books.

Evans, W. J. 1995. Effects of exercise on body composition and functional capacity of the elderly. *The Journals of Gerontology: Series A. Biological Sciences and Medical Sciences* 50(special number):147-150.

Evans, W. J. 1999. Exercise training guidelines for the elderly. *Medicine and Science in Sports and Exercise* 31(1):12-17.

Fallon, S. 1995. *Nourishing Traditions: The Cookbook That Challenges Politically Correct Nutrition and the Diet Dictocrats.* With M. G. Enig. San Diego: ProMotion Publishing.

Fallon, S., and M. G. Enig. 1999. Out of Africa: What Dr. Price and Dr. Burkitt discovered in their studies of sub-Saharan Tribes. *Price-Pottenger Nutrition Foundation Health Journal* 21(1):1-5.

Felson, D. T., Y. Zhang, M. T. Hannan, W. B. Kannel, and D. P. Kiel. 1995. Alcohol intake and bone mineral density in elderly men and women: The Framingham Study. *American Journal of Epidemiology* 142(5):485-492.

Feskanich, D., P. Weber, W. C. Willett, H. Rockett, S. L. Booth, and G. A. Colditz. 1999. Vitamin K intake and hip fractures in women: A prospective study. *American Journal of Clinical Nutrition* 69(1):74-79.

Feskanich, D., W. C. Willett, and G. A. Colditz. 2003. Calcium, vitamin D, milk consumption, and hip fractures: A prospective study among postmenopausal women. *American Journal of Clinical Nutrition* 77(2):504-511.

Feskanich, D., W. C. Willett, M. J. Stampfer, and G. A. Colditz. 1997. Milk, dietary calcium, and bone fractures in women: A 12-year prospective study. *American Journal of Public Health* 87(6):992-997.

Fields, M. 1998. Nutritional factors adversely influencing the glucose/insulin system. *Journal of the American College of Nutrition* 17(4):317-321.

Fleisher, M. A. 2006. The critical importance of dietary iodine. *Natural Awakenings, Greater Richmond Edition*, January. www.narichmond.com/critical_importance_of_dietary_iodine.html. Accessed April 25, 2008.

Fontana, L., J. L. Shew, J. O. Holloszy, and D. T. Villreal. 2005. Low bone mass in subjects on a long-term raw vegetarian diet. *Archives of Internal Medicine* 165(6):684-689.

Frankenfield, D., E. Muth, and W. A. Rowe. 1998. The Harris-Benedict studies of human basal metabolism: History and limitations. *Journal of the American Dietetic Association* 98(4):439-445.

Freeman, R. B., and R. Schettkat. 2005. Marketization of household production and the EU-US gap in work. *Economic Policy* 20(41):6-50.

Fuchs, N. K. 2003. 4 major myths about osteoporosis. *Women's Health Letter*, December.

Gaby, A. R. 1994. *Preventing and Reversing Osteoporosis.* Rocklin, CA: Prima Publishing.

García Sáenz, J. A., S. López Tarruella, B. García Paredes, L. Rodríguez Lajusticia, L. Villalobos, and E. Díaz Rubio. 2007. Osteonecrosis of the jaw as an adverse bisphosphonate event: Three cases of bone metastatic prostate cancer patients treated with zoledronic acid. *Medicina Oral, Patología Oral, y Cirugía Bucal* 12(5):E351-E356.

Geuns, J. M. 2003. Stevioside. *Phytochemistry* 64(5):913-921.

Gittleman, A. L. 1993. *Supernutrition for Menopause.* New York: Pocket Books.

Greden, J. F., B. S. Victor, P. Fontaine, and M. Lubetsky. 1980. Caffeine-withdrawal headache: A clinical profile. *Psychosomatics* 21(5):411-413, 417-418.

Greendale, G. A., E. Barrett-Connor, S. Edelstein, S. Ingles, and R. Haile. 1994. Dietary sodium and bone mineral density: Results of a 16-year follow-up study. *Journal of the American Geriatrics Society* 42(10):1050-1055.

Guardia, G., N. Parikh, T. Eskridge, E. Phillips, G. Divine, and D. S. Rao. 2008. Prevalence of vitamin D depletion among subjects seeking advice on osteoporosis: A five-year cross-sectional study with public health implications. *Osteoporosis International* 19(1):13-19.

Hallström, H., A. Wolk, A. Glynn, and K. Michaëlsson. 2006. Coffee, tea and caffeine consumption in relation to osteoporotic fracture risk in a cohort of Swedish women. *Osteoporosis International* 17(7):1055-1064.

Hands, E. 1990. *The Food Finder: Food Sources of Vitamins and Minerals.* Salem, OR: Esha Research.

Hannan, M. T., K. L. Tucker, B. Dawson-Hughes, L. A. Cupples, D. T. Felson, and D. P. Kiel. 2000. Effect of dietary protein on bone loss in elderly men and women: The Framingham Osteoporosis Study. *Journal of Bone and Mineral Research* 15(12):2504-2512.

Harrington, M., and K. D. Cashman. 2003. High salt intake appears to increase bone resorption in postmenopausal women but high potassium intake ameliorates this adverse effect. *Nutrition Reviews* 61(5 pt. 1):179-183.

Hegsted, D. M. 2001. Fractures, calcium, and the modern diet. *American Journal of Clinical Nutrition* 74(5):571-573.

Hernández-Avila, M., G. A. Colditz, M. J. Stampfer, B. Rosner, F. E. Speizer, and W. C. Willett. 1991. Caffeine, moderate alcohol intake, and risk of fractures of the hip and forearm in middle-aged women. *American Journal of Clinical Nutrition* 54(1):157-163.

Hillier, T. A., J. H. Rizzo, K. L. Pedula, K. L. Stone, J. A. Cauley, D. C. Bauer, and S. R. Cummings. 2003. Nulliparity and fracture risk in older women: The study of osteoporotic fractures. *Journal of Bone and Mineral Research* 18(5):893-899.

Holden, C., and R. Mace. 1997. Phylogenetic analysis of the evolution of lactose digestion in adults. *Human Biology* 69(5):605-628.

Holick, M. F. 2004. Sunlight and vitamin D for bone health and prevention of autoimmune diseases, cancers, and cardiovascular disease. *American Journal of Clinical Nutrition* 80(6 suppl.):1678S-1688S.

Holick, M. F., Q. Shao, W. W. Liu, and T. C. Chen. 1992. The vitamin D content of fortified milk and infant formula. *New England Journal of Medicine* 326(18)1178-1181.

Hunt, C. D., and L. K. Johnson. 2007. Calcium requirements: New estimations for men and women by cross-sectional statistical analyses of calcium balance data from metabolic studies. *American Journal of Clinical Nutrition* 86(4):1054-1063.

Hunter, B. T. 1961. *Natural Foods Cookbook.* New York: Simon & Schuster.

Institute of Medicine. 1997. *Dietary Reference Intakes: Calcium, Phosphorus, Magnesium, Vitamin D, and Fluoride.* Washington, DC: National Academy Press.

Institute of Medicine. 2004. *Dietary Reference Intakes: Water, Potassium, Sodium, Chloride, and Sulfate.* Washington, DC: National Academy Press.

International Osteoporosis Foundation. 2007. Facts and statistics about osteoporosis and its impact. www.iofbonehealth.org/facts-and-statistics.html#factsheet-category-23. Accessed February 15, 2008.

Jackson, C., S. Gaugris, S. S. Sen, and D. Hosking. 2007. The effect of cholecalciferol (vitamin $D_3$) on the risk of fall and fracture: A meta-analysis. *QJM: Monthly Journal of the Association of Physicians* 100(4):185-192.

Jacobus, C. H., M. F. Holick, Q. Shao, T. C. Chen, I. A. Holm, J. M. Kolodny, G. E. Fuleihan, and E. W. Seely. 1992. Hypervitaminosis D associated with drinking milk. *New England Journal of Medicine* 326(18):1173-1177.

Jefferson, W. N., E. Padilla-Banks, and R. R. Newbold. 2007. Disruption of the developing female reproductive system by phytoestrogens: Genistein as an example. *Molecular Nutrition and Food Research* 51(7):832-844.

Jensen, H. H., and S. T. Yen. 1996. U.S. food expenditures away from home by type of meal. *Canadian Journal of Agricultural Economics* 44:67-80.

Kanis, J. A. 1996. Estrogens, the menopause, and osteoporosis. *Bone* 19(5 suppl.):185S-190S.

Kanis, J. A. 2002. Diagnosis of osteoporosis and assessment of fracture risk. *Lancet* 359(9321):1929-1936.

Kato, Y., K. Sato, A. Sata, K. Omori, K. Nakajima, K. Tokinaga, T. Obara, and K. Takano. 2004. Hypercalcemia induced by excessive intake of calcium supplement, presenting similar findings of primary hyperparathyroidism. *Endocrine Journal* 51(6):557-562.

Kim, M. J., M. S. Shim, M. K. Kim, Y. Lee, Y. G. Shin, C. H. Chung, and S. O. Kwon. 2003. Effect of chronic alcohol ingestion on bone mineral density in males without liver cirrhosis. *Korean Journal of Internal Medicine* 18(3):174-180.

Kirschmann, G. J., and J. D. Kirschmann. 1996. *Nutrition Almanac.* 4th ed. New York: McGraw-Hill.

Klesges, R. C., K. D. Ward, M. L. Shelton, W. B. Applegate, E. D. Cantler, G. M. Palmieri, K. Harmon, and J. Davis. 1996. Changes in bone mineral content in male athletes: Mechanisms of action and intervention effects. *Journal of the American Medical Association* 276(3):226-230.

Kornfeld, M., and S. Hamanaka. 2005. *The Healthy Hedonist: More Than 200 Delectable Flexitarian Recipes for Relaxed Daily Feasts.* New York: Simon & Schuster.

Koval, K. D., and J. D. Zuckerman. 2000. *Hip Fractures: A Practical Guide to Management.* New York: Springer-Verlag.

Krieger, N. S., K. K. Frick, and D. A. Bushinsky. 2004. Mechanism of acid-induced bone resorption. *Current Opinion in Nephrology and Hypertension* 13(4):423-436.

Krupski, T. L., M. R. Smith, W. C. Lee, C. L. Pashos, J. Brandman, Q. Wang, M. Botteman, and M. S. Litwin. 2004. Natural history of bone complications in men with prostate carcinoma initiating androgen deprivation therapy. *Cancer* 101(3):541-549.

Kushi, L. H., R. M. Fee, A. R. Folsom, P. J. Mink, K. E. Anderson, and T. A. Sellers. 1997. Physical activity and mortality in postmenopausal women. *Journal of the American Medical Association* 277(16):1287-1292.

Laan, R. F., P. L. van Riel, L. B. van de Putte, L. J. van Erning, M. A. van't Hof, and J. A. Lemmens. 1993. Low-dose prednisone induces rapid reversible axial bone loss in patients with rheumatoid arthritis: A randomized, controlled study. *Annals of Internal Medicine* 119(10):963-968.

Laitinen, K., C. Lamberg-Allardt, R. Tunninen, M. Härkönen, and M. Välimäki. 1992. Bone mineral density and abstention-induced changes in bone and mineral metabolism in noncirrhotic male alcoholics. *American Journal of Medicine* 93(6):642-650.

Langlois, J. A., T. Harris, A. C. Looker, and J. Madans. 1996. Weight change between age 50 years and old age is associated with risk of hip fracture in white women aged 67 years and older. *Archives of Internal Medicine* 156(9):989-994.

Langlois, J. A., M. Visser, L. S. Davidovic, S. Maggi, G. Li, and T. B. Harris. 1998. Hip fracture risk in older white men is associated with change in body weight from age 50 years to old age. *Archives of Internal Medicine* 158(9):990-996.

Lark, S. M. 2003. *The Doctor in Your Refrigerator.* Potomac, MD: Healthy Directions.

Laugesen, M., and R. Elliott. 2003. Ischaemic heart disease, type 1 diabetes, and cow milk A1 beta-casein. *New Zealand Medical Journal* 116(1168):U295.

Lenart, B. A., D. G. Lorich, and J. M. Lane. 2008. Atypical fractures of the femoral diaphysis in postmenopausal women taking alendronate. *New England Journal of Medicine* 358(12):1304-1306.

Li, F., P. Harmer, K. J. Fisher, E. McAuley, N. Chaumeton, E. Eckstrom, and N. L. Wilson. 2005. Tai chi and fall reductions in older adults: A randomized controlled trial. *The Journals of Gerontology. Series A, Biological Sciences and Medical Sciences* 60(2):187–94.

Liebman, B. 1997. Vitamin D deficiency: The silent epidemic [interview with Michael F. Holick]. *Nutrition Action Healthletter*, January 10. www.encyclopedia.com/doc/IG1-19928282.html. Accessed April 22, 2008.

Liedloff, J. 1986. *The Continuum Concept: In Search of Happiness Lost.* Cambridge, MA: DaCapo Press.

Lim, L. S., L. J. Harnack, D. Lazovich, and A. R. Folsom. 2004. Vitamin A intake and the risk of hip fracture in postmenopausal women: The Iowa Women's Health Study. *Osteoporosis International* 15(7):552-559.

Lipski, E. 1996. *Digestive Wellness.* New Canaan, CT: Keats Publishing.

López, A. M., M. A. Pena, R. Hernández, F. Val, B. Martín, and J. A. Riancho. 2005. Fracture risk in patients with prostate cancer on androgen deprivation therapy. *Osteoporosis International* 16(6):707-711.

Lutwak, L., and L. Goulder. 1988. *The Strong Bones Diet: The High Calcium Low Calorie Way to Prevent Osteoporosis.* Gainesville, FL: Triad Publishing.

Macdonald, H. M., S. A. New, M. H. Golden, M. K. Campbell, and D. M. Reid. 2004. Nutritional associations with bone loss during the menopausal transition: Evidence of a beneficial effect of calcium, alcohol, and fruit and vegetable nutrients and of a detrimental effect of fatty acids. *American Journal of Clinical Nutrition* 79(1):155-165.

Madhok, R., L. J. Melton III, E. J. Atkinson, W. M. O'Fallon, and D. G. Lewallen. 1993. Urban vs rural increase in hip fracture incidence: Age and sex of 901 cases 1980-89 in Olmsted County, U.S.A. *Acta Orthopaedica Scandinavica* 64(5):543-548.

Malatesta, M., C. Caporaloni, S. Gavaudan, M. B. Rocchi, S. Serafini, C. Tiberi, and G. Ganzanelli. 2002. Ultrastructural morphometrical and immunocytochemical analyses of hepatocyte nuclei from mice fed on genetically modified soybean. *Cell Structure and Function* 27(4):173-180.

Malatesta, M., C. Caporaloni, L. Rossi, S. Battistelli, M. B. Rocchi, F. Tonucci, and G. Gazzanelli. 2002. Ultrastructural analysis of pancreatic acinar cells from mice fed on genetically modified soybean. *Journal of Anatomy* 201(5):409-415.

Masterjohn, C. 2006. From seafood to sunshine: A new understanding of vitamin D safety. *Wise Traditions in Food, Farming, and the Healing Arts* Fall: 14-33.

May, H., R. Reader, S. Murphy, and K. T. Khaw. 1995. Self-reported tooth loss and bone mineral density in older men and women. *Age and Ageing* 24(3):217-221.

Mayo Clinic. 2007. Osteoporosis: Prevention. www.mayoclinic.com/health/osteoporosis/DS00128/DSECTION=9. Accessed April 5, 2008.

McCrory, M. A., P. J. Fuss, E. Saltzman, and S. B. Roberts. 2000. Dietary determinants of energy intake and weight regulation in healthy adults. *Journal of Nutrition* 130(2S suppl.):276S-279S.

Melton, L. J., III, C. S. Crowson, and W. M. O'Fallon. 1999. Fracture incidence in Olmsted County, Minnesota: Comparison of urban with rural rates and changes in urban rates over time. *Osteoporosis International* 9(1):29-37.

Mercola, J. 2005. What you don't know about fluoridation could hurt you. http://articles.mercola.com/sites/articles/archive/2005/08/02/fluoridation-part-four.aspx. Accessed April 20, 2008.

Meyer, H. E., J. I. Pedersen, E. B. Loken, and A. Tverdal. 1997. Dietary factors and the incidence of hip fracture in middle-aged Norwegians: A prospective study. *American Journal of Epidemiology* 145(2):117-123.

Miggiano, G. A., and L. Gagliardi. 2005. Diet, nutrition and bone health. [In Italian.] *Clinica Terapeutica* 156(1-2):47-56.

Miller, D. W., Jr. 2005. Fluoride follies. www.lewrockwell.com/miller/miller17.html. Accessed April 21, 2008.

Mohammad, A. R., M. Brunsvold, and R. Bauer. 1996. The strength of association between systemic postmenopausal osteoporosis and periodontal disease. *International Journal of Prosthodontics* 9(5):479-483.

Nainggolan, L. 2008. Calcium supplements increase vascular events? www.medscape.com/viewarticle/569160. Accessed April 21, 2008.

Nakamura, K. M. Nashimoto, Y. Okuda, T. Ota, and M. Yamamoto. 2002. Fish as a major source of vitamin D in the Japanese diet. *Nutrition* 18(5):415-416.

National Institutes of Health Consensus Conference. 1994. Optimal calcium intake: Consensus Development Panel on Optimal Calcium Intake. *Journal of the American Medical Association* 272(24):1942-1948.

National Osteoporosis Foundation. 2008a. Fast facts. www.nof.org/osteoporosis/diseasefacts.htm. Accessed February 15, 2008.

National Osteoporosis Foundation. 2008b. Prevention. www.nof.org/prevention/index.htm. Accessed April 5, 2008.

National Women's Health Network. 2008. Osteoporosis Fact Sheet. www.nwhn.org.

Nesse, R. M., and G. C. Williams. 1994. *Why We Get Sick: The New Science of Darwinian Medicine.* New York: Vintage Books.

Nicklas, T. A., T. Baranowski, K. W. Cullen, and G. Berenson. 2001. Eating patterns, dietary quality and obesity. *Journal of the American College of Nutrition* 20(6):599-608.

Nieves, J. W. 2005. Osteoporosis: The role of micronutrients. *American Journal of Clinical Nutrition* 81(5):1232S-1239S.

Nnakwe, N., and C. A. Kies. 1985. Mouse bone composition and breaking strength: Effects of varying calcium and phosphorus content in animal or plant protein diets. In *Nutritional Bioavailability of Calcium*, ed. C. A. Kies. Washington, DC: American Chemical Society.

Nordin, B. C. 2000. Calcium requirement is a sliding scale. *American Journal of Clinical Nutrition* 71(6):1381-1383.

Northrup, C. 1998. *Women's Bodies, Women's Wisdom: Creating Physical and Emotional Health and Healing.* New York: Bantam Doubleday Dell.

Northrup, C. 2006. *The Wisdom of Menopause.* New York: Bantam.

Northwestern University. 2007. Nutrition fact sheet: Vitamin A. 2007. www.feinberg.northwestern.edu/nutrition/factsheets/vitamin-a.html. Accessed April 5, 2008.

Ojeda, L. 1995. *Menopause Without Medicine.* Alameda, CA: Hunter House.

Ott, S. M. 1993a. Clinical effects of bisphosphonates in involutional osteoporosis. *Journal of Bone and Mineral Research* 8(suppl. 2):S597-S606.

Ott, S. M. 1993b. When bone mass fails to predict bone failure. *Calcified Tissue International* 53(suppl. 1):S7-S13.

Ott, S. M. 1994. Bone mass measurements: Reasons to be cautious. *British Medical Journal* 308(6934):931-932.

Ott, S. M. 2004. Diet for the heart or the bone: A biological tradeoff. *American Journal of Clinical Nutrition* 79(1):4-5.

Outila, T. A., P. H. Mattila, V. I. Piironen, and C. J. Lamberg-Allerdt. 1999. Bioavailability of vitamin D from wild edible mushrooms (*Cantharellus tubaeformis*) as measured with a human bioassay. *American Journal of Clinical Nutrition* 69(1):95-98.

Parker-Pope, T. 2008. Drugs to build bones may weaken them. *New York Times*, July 15. www.nytimes.com/2008/07/15/health/15well.html. Accessed July 15, 2008.

Pearson, D., and L. McTaggart. 1996. Osteoporosis: A load of old bones. *What Doctors Don't Tell You* 6(12):2-3. Available in part at www.healthy.net/scr/article.asp?Id=3140. Accessed April 21, 2008.

Pickering, G. W. 1956. The purpose of medical education. *British Medical Journal* 2(4985):113-116.

Price, W. 1979. *Nutrition and Physical Degeneration.* La Mesa, CA: Price-Pottenger Nutrition Foundation.

Prior, I. A., F. Davidson, C. E. Salmond, and Z. Czochanska. 1981. Cholesterol, coconuts, and diet on Polynesian atolls: A natural experiment: The Pukapuka and Tokelau island studies. *American Journal of Clinical Nutrition* 34(8):1552-1561.

Quandt, S. A., J. G. Spangler, L. D. Case, R. A. Bell, and A. E. Belflower. 2005. Smokeless tobacco use accelerates age-related loss of bone mineral density among older women in a multi-ethnic rural community. *Journal of Cross-Cultural Gerontology* 20(2):109-125.

Ravnskov, U. 2000. *The Cholesterol Myths: Exposing the Fallacy That Saturated Fat and Cholesterol Cause Heart Disease.* Washington, DC: New Trends Publishing.

Reichrath, J. 2006. The challenge resulting from positive and negative effects of sunlight: How much solar UV exposure is appropriate to balance between risks of vitamin D deficiency and skin cancer? *Progress in Biophysics and Molecular Biology* 92(1):9-16.

Rossouw, J. E., G. L. Anderson, R. L. Prentice, A. Z. LaCroix, C. Kooperberg, M. L. Stefanick, R. D. Jackson, S. A. Beresford, B. V. Howard, K. C. Johnson, J. M. Kitchen, and J. Ockene. 2002. Risks and benefits of estrogen plus progestin in healthy postmenopausal women: Principal results from the Women's Health Initiative randomized controlled trial. *Journal of the American Medical Association* 288(3):321-333.

Roughead, Z. K., J. R. Hunt, L. K. Johnson, T. M. Badger, and G. I. Lykken. 2005. Controlled substitution of soy protein for meat protein: Effects on calcium retention, bone, and cardiovascular health indices in postmenopausal women. *Journal of Clinical Endocrinology and Metabolism* 90(1):181-189.

Roughead, Z. K., L. K. Johnson, G. I. Lykken, and J. R. Hunt. 2003. Controlled high meat diets do not affect calcium retention or indices of bone status in healthy postmenopausal women. *Journal of Nutrition* 133(4):1020-1026.

Ruggiero, S. L., and S. J. Drew. 2007. Osteonecrosis of the jaws and bisphosphonate therapy. *Journal of Dental Research* 86(11):1013-1021.

Runowicz, C. 2003. Hormone therapy: When and for how long? *HealthNews* 9(2):1-2.

Rylander, R., T. Remer, S. Berkemeyer, and J. Vormann. 2006. Acid-base status affects renal magnesium losses in healthy, elderly persons. *Journal of Nutrition* 136(9):2374-2377.

Sanson, G. 2003. *The Myth of Osteoporosis: What Every Woman Should Know About Creating Bone Health.* Ann Arbor, MI: MCD Publications.

Schepers, A. R. 2007. Beyond the sugar bowl: Sweeteners closer to Mother Nature. *Environmental Nutrition* 30(6):2.

Seely, S. 2002. The connection between milk and mortality from coronary heart disease. *Journal of Epidemiology and Community Health* 56(12):958.

Severson, K. 2005. Harlem school introduces children to Swiss chard. *New York Times*, September 9. www.nytimes.com/2005/09/09/nyregion/09promise.html. Accessed April 5, 2008.

Shaw, C. K. 1993. An epidemiologic study of osteoporosis in Taiwan. *Annals of Epidemiology* 3(3):264-271.

Sheldon, T. 2001. NHS CRD founding director clarifies results of York fluoridation review. www.fluoridealert.org/sheldon.htm. Accessed May 16, 2008.

Shikany, J. M., and G. L. White Jr. 2000. Dietary guidelines for chronic disease prevention. *Southern Medical Journal* 93(12):1138-1151.

Shils, M. E., J. A. Olson, M. Shike, and A. C. Ross, eds. 1994. *Modern Nutrition in Health and Disease.* Philadelphia: Lea & Febiger.

Shumaker, S. A., C. Legault, S. R. Rapp, L. Thal, R. B. Wallace, J. K. Ockene, S. L. Hendrix, B. N. Jones III, A. R. Assaf, R. D. Jackson, J. M. Kotchen, S. Wassertheil-Smoller, and J. Wactawski-Wende. 2003. Estrogen plus progestin and the incidence of dementia and mild cognitive impairment in postmenopausal women: The Women's Health Initiative Memory Study: A randomized controlled trial. *Journal of the American Medical Association* 289(20):2651-2662.

Silverman, K., S. M. Evans, E. C. Strain, and R. R. Griffiths. 1992. Withdrawal syndrome after the double-blind cessation of caffeine consumption. *New England Journal of Medicine* 327(16):1109-1114.

Smith, J. M. 2007. *Genetic Roulette: The Documented Health Risks of Genetically Engineered Foods.* Fairfield, IA: Yes! Books.

Snyder, B. D., D. A. Hauser-Kara, J. A. Hipp, D. Zurakowski, A. C. Hecht, and M. C. Gebhardt. 2006. Predicting fracture through benign skeletal lesions with quantitative computed tomography. *Journal of Bone and Joint Surgery: American Volume* 88(1):55-70.

Society for Neuroscience. 2003. Sugar addiction. *Brain Briefings*, October. www.sfn.org/index.cfm?pagename=brainBriefings_sugarAddiction. Accessed April 24, 2008.

Song, J., X. Hu, M. Shi, M. A. Knepper, and C. A. Ecelbarger. 2004. Effects of dietary fat, NaCl, and fructose on renal sodium and water transporter abundances and systemic blood pressure. *American Journal of Physiology: Renal Physiology* 287(6):F1204-F1212.

Spencer, H., and L. Kramer. 1985. Osteoporosis: Calcium, fluoride, and aluminum interactions. *Journal of the American College of Nutrition* 4(1):121-128.

Spencer, H., and L. Kramer. 1987. Osteoporosis, calcium requirement, and factors causing calcium loss. *Clinics in Geriatric Medicine* 3(2):389-402.

Spencer, H., L. Kramer, M. DeBartolo, C. Norris, and D. Osis. 1983. Further studies of the effect of a high protein diet as meat on calcium metabolism. *American Journal of Clinical Nutrition* 37(6):924-929.

Tan, T. 2005. Drugs for prostate cancer. *What Doctors Don't Tell You* 16(1):7. Available in part at www.wddty.com/033638003712728997845/drugs-for-prostate-cancer.html. Accessed April 22, 2008.

Thomas, W. J. 1994. Exercise, age, and the bones. *Southern Medical Journal* 87(4):S23-S25.

Thompson, C. 2007. Why New Yorkers last longer. *New York Magazine*, August 13.

Tjäderhane, L., and M. Larmas. 1998. A high sucrose diet decreases the mechanical strength of bones in growing rats. *Journal of Nutrition* 128(10):1807-1810.

Tsukahara, J., A. Toda, J. Goto, and I. Ezawa. 1994. Cross-sectional and longitudinal studies on the effect of water exercise in controlling bone loss in Japanese post-menopausal women. *Journal of Nutritional Science and Vitaminology (Tokyo)* 40(1):37-47.

Tuck, S. P., and R. M. Francis. 2002. Osteoporosis. *Postgraduate Medical Journal* 78(923):526-532.

Tufts University. 1997. Like to walk? Put away your walking shoes. *Tufts University Health and Nutrition Letter* 15:1.

U.S. Food and Drug Administration. 2008. Information on bisphosphonates (marketed as Actonel, Actonel+Ca, Aredia, Boniva, Didronel, Fosamax, Fosamax+D, Reclast, Skelid, and Zometa). www.fda.gov/cder/drug/infopage/bisphosphonates/default.htm. Accessed February 28, 2008.

Utsumi, M., C. Azuma, S. Tohno, Y. Tohno, Y. Moriwake, T. Minami, and M. O. Yamada. 2005. Increases of calcium and magnesium and decrease of iron in human posterior longitudinal ligaments of the cervical spine with aging. *Biological Trace Elements Research* 103(3):217-228.

Van der Rhee, H. J., E. de Vries, and J. W. Coebergh. 2007. Favourable and unfavourable effects of exposure to sunlight. [In Dutch.] *Nederlands Tijdschrift voor Geneeskunde* 151(2):118-122.

Vasquez, A., G. Manso, and J. Cannell. 2004. The clinical importance of vitamin D (cholecalciferol): A paradigm shift with implications for all healthcare providers. *Alternative Therapies in Health and Medicine* 10(5):28-36; quiz 37, 94.

Vecchio, L., B. Cisterna, M. Malatesta, T. E. Martin, and M. Biggiogera. 2004. Ultrastructural analysis of testes from mice fed on genetically modified soybean. *European Journal of Histochemistry* 48(4):448-454.

Victor, B. S., M. Lubetsky, and J. F. Greden. 1981. Somatic manifestations of caffeinism. *Journal of Clinical Psychiatry* 42(5):185-188.

Vilela, M. L., E. Willingham, J. Buckley, B. C. Liu, K. Agras, Y. Shiroyanagi, and L. S. Baskin. 2007. Endocrine disruptors and hypospadias: Role of genistein and the fungicide vinclozolin. *Urology* 70(3):618-621.

Vollmer, R. T. 2007. Solar elastosis in cutaneous melanoma. *American Journal of Clinical Pathology* 128(2):260-264.

Wade, N. 2005. Your body is younger than you think. *New York Times*, August 2. www.nytimes.com/2005/08/02/science/02cell.html. Accessed April 5, 2008.

Waldrop, M. M. 1992. *Complexity: The Emerging Science at the Edge of Order and Chaos.* New York and London: Simon & Schuster.

Ward, K. D., and R. C. Klesges. 2001. A meta-analysis of the effects of cigarette smoking on bone mineral density. *Calcified Tissue International* 68(5):259-270.

Watkins, T. R., K. Pandya, and O. Mickelson. 1985. Urinary acid and calcium excretion: Effect of soy versus meat in human diets. In *Nutritional Bioavailability of Calcium*, ed. C. A. Kies. Washington, DC: American Chemical Society.

Wells, P. 1989. *Bistro Cooking.* New York: Workman.

Wengreen, H. J., R. G. Munger, N. A. West, D. R. Cutler, C. D. Corcoran, J. Zhang, and N. E. Sassano. 2004. Dietary protein intake and risk of osteoporotic hip fracture in elderly residents of Utah. *Journal of Bone and Mineral Research* 19(4):537-545.

White, S. C., K. A. Atchison, J. A. Gornbein, A. Nattiv, A. Paganini-Hill, and S. K. Service. 2006. Risk factors for fractures in older men and women: The Leisure World Cohort Study. *Gender Medicine* 3(2):110-123.

Whitney, E., and S. R. Rolfes. 2005. *Understanding Nutrition.* Belmont, CA: Thomson Wadsworth.

Wilford, J. N. 1997. Volcano captured corn, chilies and house mice. *New York Times*, April 8. http://query.nytimes.com/gst/fullpage.html?res=9F0DEFDA1F3DF93B A35757C0A961958260. Accessed April 5, 2008.

Williams, S. 1996. Caffeine in your decaf? *Self* 18(3).

Williamson, C. S. 2007. Is organic food better for our health? *Nutrition Bulletin* 32(2):104-108.

Wilson, E. E., A. Awonusi, M. D. Morris, D. H. Kohn, M. M. Tecklenburg, and L. W. Beck. 2005. Highly ordered interstitial water observed in bone by nuclear magnetic resonance. *Journal of Bone and Mineral Research* 20(4):625-634.

Winter, R. 1995. *A Consumer's Guide to Medicines in Food.* New York: Crown Trade Paperbacks.

Wong, P. K., J. J. Christie, and J. D. Wark. 2007. The effects of smoking on bone health. *Clinical Science* (London) 113(5):233-241.

World Health Organization. 2003. *Prevention and Management of Osteoporosis: Report of a WHO Scientific Group.* Technical Report Series, no. 921. Geneva: World Health Organization.

Worthington, V. 1998. Effect of agricultural methods on nutritional quality: A comparison of organic with conventional crops. *Alternative Therapies in Health and Medicine* 4(1):58-69.

Wuttke, W., H. Jarry, and D. Seidlová-Wuttke. 2007. Isoflavones: Safe food additives or dangerous drugs? *Ageing Research Reviews* 6(2):150-188.

Wylie-Rosett, J., C. J. Segal-Isaacson, and A. Segal-Isaacson. 2004. Carbohydrates and increases in obesity: Does the type of carbohydrate make a difference? *Obesity Research* 12(suppl. 2):124S-129S.

Yudkin, J. 1972. *Pure, White, and Deadly: The Problem of Sugar.* London: Davis-Poynter.

Zaloga, G. P., K. A. Harvey, W. Stillwell, and R. Siddiqui. 2006. Trans fatty acids and coronary heart disease. *Nutrition in Clinical Practice* 21(5):505-512.

Annemarie Colbin, Ph.D., is a health educator and award-winning writer, consultant, and lecturer. She is the founder and CEO of the Natural Gourmet Institute for Health and Culinary Arts in New York City, which offers a licensed and accredited career program in natural foods cuisine. The associated Natural Gourmet Institute for Food and Health offers avocational classes in health-supportive cooking and natural healing to the general public. Colbin has also taught at several New York City schools, including the Institute for Integrative Nutrition, the New York City Open Center, Touro College, and Empire State College. She is author of several books including *Food and Healing* and writes a column, "Food and Your Health," for *New York Spirit* magazine. Colbin offers private wellness consultations. She lives in New York City with her husband, journalist Bernard Gavzer. You can learn more about the Natural Gourmet Institute for Health and Culinary Arts at www.naturalgourmetinstitute.com.

Foreword author **Mark Hyman, MD**, is coauthor of *The Detox Box* and the best-selling *Ultraprevention*. He is editor-in-chief of *Alternative Therapies in Health and Medicine*, the most prestigious journal in the field of integrative medicine. Hyman lives in western Massachusetts.

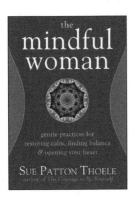
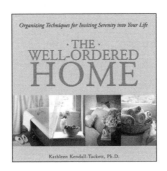
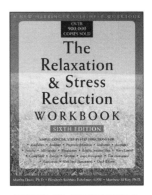
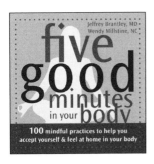
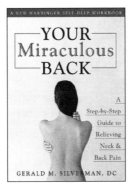
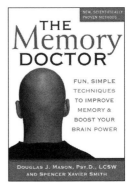